Performance and the Medical Body

Performance and Science: Interdisciplinary Dialogues explores the interactions between science and performance, providing readers with a unique guide to current practices and research in this fast-expanding field. Through shared themes and case studies, the series offers rigorous vocabularies and methods for empirical studies of performance, with each volume involving collaboration between performance scholars, practitioners and scientists. The series encompasses the modalities of performance to include drama, dance and music.

SERIES EDITORS

John Lutterbie

Chair of the Departments of Art and of Theatre Arts at Stony Brook University, USA

Nicola Shaughnessy

Professor of Performance at the University of Kent, UK

IN THE SAME SERIES

Performance and the Medical Body

Edited by Alex Mermikides and Gianna Bouchard

Bloomsbury Methuen Drama
An imprint of Bloomsbury Publishing Plc

B L O O M S B U R Y
LONDON · OXFORD · NEW YORK · NEW DELHI · SYDNEY

Bloomsbury Methuen Drama

An imprint of Bloomsbury Publishing Plc

Imprint previously known as Methuen Drama

50 Bedford Square	1385 Broadway
London	New York
WC1B 3DP	NY 10018
UK	USA

www.bloomsbury.com

**BLOOMSBURY, METHUEN DRAMA and the Diana logo are trademarks of
Bloomsbury Publishing Plc**

First published 2016

British Library Cataloguing-in-Publication Data
A catalogue record for this book is available from the British Library.

ISBN: HB: 978-1-4725-7078-9
ePDF: 978-1-4725-7080-2
ePub: 978-1-4725-7079-6

Library of Congress Cataloging-in-Publication Data
A catalog record for this book is available from the Library of Congress.

Typeset by Integra Software Services Pvt. Ltd
Printed and bound in Great Britain

CONTENTS

LIST OF
ILLUSTRATIONS

LIST OF
CONTRIBUTORS

Gianna Bouchard is Principal Lecturer in Drama at Anglia Ruskin University, Cambridge, UK. Her research focuses on contemporary performance and live art in relation to medical science. She is co-editor of 'On Medicine', a special issue of *Performance Research* (2014), and her work has been published in various edited collections and journals, including *Contemporary Theatre Review* and *Performance Research*.

Emma Brodzinski is a Senior Lecturer in drama and theatre at Royal Holloway, University of London. She has research interests in contemporary theatre practice and has previously published a range of work covering theatre in health, theatre and therapy, devising and mainstream performance. She also works as a dramatherapist.

Professor Gabriella Giannachi is Professor of Performance and New Media at the University of Exeter, UK. She has published a number of books including *Virtual Theatres* (2004); *The Politics of New Media Theatre* (2007); *Performing Presence: Between the Live and the Simulated*, co-authored with Nick Kaye (2011); *Performing Mixed Reality*, co-authored with Steve Benford (2011); and *Archaeologies of Presence*, co-edited with Michael Shanks and Nick Kaye. She has written papers for a number of humanities and science journals, and has been involved in a number of AHRC and RCUK funded projects in collaboration with Tate, Royal Albert Memorial Museum and Art Gallery, 1010 Media and Exeter City Football Club Supporters Trust.

Professor **Roger Kneebone** is Professor of Surgical Education and Engagement Science at Imperial College, London, and jointly directs the Imperial College Centre for Engagement and Simulation Science. His innovative work on contextualized simulation builds on his personal experience as a surgeon and a general practitioner, and his interest in domains of expertise beyond medicine. He sees engagement as a translational resource, which bridges the worlds of clinical practice, biomedical science, patients and society. Roger leads an unorthodox and creative team of clinicians, computer scientists, artists, social scientists and performers. He has an international profile as an academic and innovator and is a Wellcome Trust Engagement Fellow.

Professor **Petra Kuppers** is a disability culture activist, a community performance artist and a Professor at the University of Michigan. She also teaches on Goddard College's Low Residency MFA in Interdisciplinary Arts. She leads The Olimpias, a performance research collective (www.olimpias.org). Her *Disability Culture and Community Performance: Find a Strange and Twisted Shape* (Palgrave, 2011; paperback 2013) explores The Olimpias' arts-based research methods. She is the author of a recent textbook *Studying Disability Arts and Culture: An Introduction* (Palgrave, 2014). Her books include *Disability and Contemporary Performance: Bodies on Edge* (Routledge, 2003), *The Scar of Visibility: Medical Performance and Contemporary Art* (Minnesota, 2007) and *Community Performance: An Introduction* (Routledge, 2007). Edited work includes *Somatic Engagement* (2011) and *Community Performance: A Reader* (2007).

P. Solomon Lennox is Lecturer in Performing Arts at Northumbria University, UK. His research work uses performance ethnography methodologies to examine the performance of identity amongst combat athletes. Focusing on amateur and professional boxers, Lennox has explored the relationship between narratives and performance practices in the formation and presentation of gendered identity. He is currently engaged in an ethnographic study of mixed martial arts (MMA), investigating the impact spaces and sites have on the narrative identities available to combat athletes. His work covers topics such as, sensuous ethnographies, somatic bodily practices, narrative performance, performance studies and performative social sciences.

Brian Lobel is a Senior Lecturer at the University of Chichester and a performer and curator who creates work about bodies and how they are watched, policed, prodded and loved by others. Projects include *BALL & Other Funny Stories About Cancer, Purge, Carpe Minuta Prima* and *Fun with Cancer Patients*. Lobel shows work internationally in a range of contexts, from medical schools to museums, marketplaces to forests, blending provocative humour with insightful reflection. Brian's work appears in an array of publications including journal articles, scripts and artist DVDs. He is a core artist with Forest Fringe and a Wellcome Trust Public Engagement Fellow.

Alex Mermikides is Senior Lecturer in Drama at Kingston University, London, UK. Her research interest is in contemporary performance-making, with a particular focus on science-engaged devised performance. Her publications include *Devising in Process* (Palgrave, 2010, co-edited with Jackie Smart), and papers in other collections. Her practice encompasses directing, performance writing and dramaturgy. Her recent production, *bloodlines*, was produced at the Science Museum, London, Antwerp University Hospital and elsewhere.

Martin O'Brien is an artist and a theorist whose performance and research draws upon his experience of suffering from cystic fibrosis. His work is concerned with physical endurance, disgust, long durations and pain-based practices to address a politics of the sick queer body and examine what it means to be born with a life-threatening disease, politically and philosophically. He has performed throughout the world, both solo and in collaboration with the pioneering performance artist Sheree Rose. He is co-editor of a special edition of Performance Research *On Medicine* and has published essays in a variety of books and journals.

Professor Jennifer Parker-Starbuck is Professor and Head of the Department of Drama, Theatre and Performance at the University of Roehampton, London. She is the author of *Cyborg Theatre: Corporeal/Technological Intersections in Multimedia Performance* (Palgrave Macmillan, 2011; paperback 2014) and co-editor with Lourdes Orozco of *Performing Animality: Animals in Performance Practice* (Palgrave, 2015). Her recent work explores animality, technology and performance and her essay 'Animal Ontologies and Media Representations: Robotics, Puppets, and the Real of War Horse' (*Theatre Journal,* Vol. 65, Number 3, October 2013) received the ATHE 2014 Outstanding Article award. She is the incoming co-editor of *Theatre Journal.*

Fiona Pettit is an independent researcher. Her current work is situated betwixt the boundaries of medical humanities and performance studies, focusing specifically on the lived experiences of people with invisible chronic illness. Earlier work examined the late nineteenth-century representations of human 'freak' exhibitions, as they were documented in medical and scientific journals, exploring the multifarious representations of human 'freak' exhibitions and the adjustments made in their depictions for varying audiences. More recently, Pettit has demonstrated how the legacy of nineteenth-century popular freak show discourse is present within the twenty-first-century *X-Men* films.

Helen Pynor is an artist whose practise explores philosophically and experientially precarious zones such as the life–death border. Her work is informed by in-depth residencies in scientific and clinical institutions, most recently the Max Planck Institute for Molecular Cell Biology and Genetics, Dresden, and the Heart and Lung Transplant Unit, St Vincent's Hospital, Sydney. Pynor's work has been exhibited widely internationally including at Ars Electronica, Science Gallery Dublin, National Centre for Contemporary Art (Russia), Australian Centre for Photography, National Taiwan Museum of Fine Arts and Wellcome Collection. Pynor holds a Bachelor of Visual Arts, a Bachelor of Science and a practice-based PhD.

Kirsten E. Shepherd-Barr is on the Faculty of English at the University of Oxford and a Fellow of St Catherine's College. She is the author of *Theatre and Evolution from Ibsen to Beckett* (2015), *Science on Stage: From Doctor Faustus to Copenhagen* (2006; paperback 2012) and *Ibsen and Early Modernist Theatre, 1890–1900* (1997). She is also co-editor of two special issues of the journal *Interdisciplinary Science Reviews* on 'New Directions in Theatre and Science' (2013 and 2014).

Suzy Willson co-founded Clod Ensemble with musician Paul Clark in 1995 and has directed all of their productions to date, including *Zero* (Sadler's Wells, 2013), *Silver Swan* (Tate Modern Turbine Hall, 2012), *Red Ladies* (Southbank Centre, 2014), *Under Glass* (Sadler's Wells and UK Tour, 2009). She also leads the company's *Performing Medicine* project and is an honorary senior lecturer at Barts and The London School of Medicine. For further information, please see: www.clodensemble.com and www.performingmedicine.com

ACKNOWLEDGEMENTS

A collection such as this would not be possible without the generosity and patience of our contributors, so thank you for making this such a stimulating and interesting project. Special thanks go to Professor Nicola Shaughnessy, for supporting the project from its very early stages, and to Professor John Lutterbie, our series editors, and to Mark Dudgeon, Emily Hockley and all at Bloomsbury Methuen Drama who helped bring it to fruition. We would also like to express our gratitude to colleagues and students at Kingston University and Anglia Ruskin University, who helped develop our understanding and enthusiasm for performance, the body and/or medicine. We have also benefitted from a range of formal and informal discussions along the way and we hope that these continue over the coming months and years, as they are the sustenance and inspiration for our work.

Finally, warmest appreciation to our families and loved ones for supporting and encouraging us. Alex thanks Olga Mermikides and Matt, Maxi and Charlie Urmenyi. Gianna thanks Paul Jackson, Judith Bouchard, Rick Burroughs, Kathryn, Alan, William and Ava Truswell, Gill Palin, and Sam and Hannah Jackson. Both Alex and Gianna dedicate the volume to their late fathers, Michael Mermikides and Alan Bouchard.

Kirsten Shepherd-Barr is indebted to Dr Sos Eltis for her careful reading of her chapter in draft form and for her excellent suggestions as to its improvement.

Roger Kneebone gratefully acknowledges the support of Wellcome Trust, Imperial College London, London Deanery (STeLI) and numerous colleagues both within and beyond Imperial. He is especially indebted to Gunther Kress (Institute of Education) and Fernando Bello (Imperial College London and co-director of ICCESS) for their collaboration around concepts of simulation, engagement and reciprocal illumination. Imperial

College Centre for Engagement and Simulation Science (ICCESS) is an unorthodox and multidisciplinary team which includes clinicians, educationalists, computer scientists, engineers, social scientists, artists and performers.

Helen Pynor's chapter in this volume is a modified version of an essay originally published in Wilson, B., Hawkins, B. and Sim, S. (2014). *Art, Science and Cultural Understanding*, Champaign, Illinois: Common Ground, pp. 189–206.

Alex Mermikides' chapter, and the volume as a whole, was inspired by a research network project supported by the Arts and Humanities Research Council under the Science in Culture theme (AH/K003518/1).

Gabriella Giannachi gratefully acknowledges the RCUK-funded Horizon Digital Economy (EP/G065802/1) for funding her research for this article, and Lynn Hershman Leeson for generously making time to explain her work.

Introduction

Alex Mermikides and Gianna Bouchard

It is hard to identify an area of our lives, at the start of the twenty-first century, where medical science does not have some kind of influence or impact. From evaluating what we eat, to getting vaccinations for holidays, from allergies to terminal illness, our cultural landscape is dominated by the medical; its policies, practices and ideologies are part and parcel of our understanding of the world. In the UK, for example, the media is saturated with stories of our National Health Service being in crisis; the spiralling cost of drugs and their continued efficacy; the impact of lifestyle on our health and well-being; our ageing population and its cost (socially and economically); and the list goes on. Its dominance in the news media is paralleled by an extraordinary abundance of television programmes, from factual documentaries, to medical reality shows and fictional soap operas set in hospitals. This fascination with the medical is nothing new and it shifts according to our social, cultural and political concerns in a certain historical moment. It also often gets focused through the latest medico-scientific 'breakthroughs', so, for instance, in the 1990s, we were particularly intrigued and challenged by cloning technologies and advances, which emerged very forcefully and with seemingly huge potentials for catastrophe or productive creativity.

Perhaps it is this vitality and prevalence of medicine in society and culture that has incited a newfound and burgeoning interest in the intersections between medicine and performance practice.

Performance and the Medical Body brings together a collection of essays that interrogate these relations. Emerging from a range of perspectives and utilizing different concepts of 'performance', the essays offer an insight into this interface, as it is being thought and practiced in the early twenty-first century. Our introduction provides some context to this social and cultural milieu and the apparent turn towards a more explicit forging of links between medicine and performance in the contemporary moment. We begin by pinpointing some historical moments of convergence between these two domains and their relationships to the body.

Looking at bodies

Maaike Bleeker has identified the theatre as a 'vision machine' and, in many ways, this same designation can be applied to modern conceptions of medicine and how it engages with its subject, the body (Bleeker, 2011). Both medicine and performance look at bodies to construct knowledge, and both are informed by various ideological framings that shape, influence and even distort those displays and their interpretation. Such explicit connections between seeing and knowing emerged in medicine from the fifteenth century onwards – the era usually identified as initiating the birth of modern medicine. Up until the early modern period, medical knowledge and practice was predicated on ancient Greek texts, which were taken as the source of all authoritative 'scientific' knowledge. An interesting example of this dependence on ancient scholarship can be found in the early demonstrations of anatomical dissection. Up until the early modern period, the body was dissected according to the work of Galen, whose writings guided the procedures and meant that the body was transformed into an illustrative prop for ancient medical ideas. These practices were then radically overturned with the arrival of Andreas Vesalius as Professor of Surgery and Anatomy at the medical school of the University of Padua in 1537 (see Cunningham, 2010). Renowned for his work as a dissector, he employed these skills to undertake dissections himself and to look to the body to locate its own 'truths' and subsequent knowledge. This new form of looking, or 'autopsia' (looking for oneself), had a fundamental impact on how medicine engaged with bodies; since the fifteenth century and Vesalius' work, 'a plethora of visual and representational instruments have been developed to help obtain new views on, and convey new insights into, human physiology' (van Dijck, 2005, 4).

Perhaps the most significant identification of a radical paradigm shift in medicine came from the French philosopher Michel Foucault. In *The Birth of the Clinic: An Archaeology of Medical Perception*, he suggests that the French Revolution (1789–1799) had a profound effect on medical practice and thought, particularly via Parisian healthcare. Developing the concept of 'anatomo-politics', Foucault argues that at this historical moment, bodies became subject to industrialization and were reconfigured as requiring disciplining and surveillance to become docile and productive:

> One of these poles – the first to be formed, it seems – centered on the body as a machine: its disciplining, the optimization of its capabilities, the extortion of its forces, the parallel increase of its usefulness and its docility, its integration into systems of efficient and economic controls, all this was ensured by the procedures of power that characterized the *disciplines*: an *anatomo-politics of the human body*. (Foucault, 1978, 139)

Previous ideas and practices from the Greco-Roman period were, at last, overturned, along with humoral medicine, in favour of an empiricist approach to medical care. This meant the development of standardized techniques of assessment, diagnosis and treatment, forging new relations between doctors and patients. The 'birth of the clinic' in Paris at the time of the revolution offered medics an unparalleled opportunity to examine and consider multitudes of patients. Not only treatments were standardized but also medical training and knowledge was transformed through the implementation of more uniform medical curricula and examinations. Doctors were now involved in direct examination of their patients' bodies, where previously symptoms were only discussed and surgeons were the only men to come into express contact with the unwell. To understand disease, pathological anatomy became crucial, in Foucault's terms, to compare with the living specimens of illness.

A central aspect of Foucault's work was in his theorization of what he called the 'medical gaze'. If, as art historian James Elkins claims, 'there is no such thing as just looking', then this medical gaze is particularly problematic (Elkins, 1996, 31). Again, Foucault argues for a distinctive paradigm at this historical moment of the French Revolution:

> … the medical gaze was also organized in a new way. First, it was no longer the gaze of any observer, but that of a doctor supported and justified by an institution, that of a doctor endowed with the power of decision and intervention. […] it was a gaze that was not content to observe what was self-evident; it must make it possible to outline chances and risks; it was calculating. (Foucault, 1973, 89)

The idea of this medical gaze and its intrinsic need to analyse, evaluate and objectify the body has become an important conceptual tool in studies of medicine, health and illness. Some of the work in this book is interested, for example, in how performance might resist and challenge this embedded sense of clinical judgement and objectification. Some also argue that the medical gaze, with its disciplinary mechanisms and interventions, is necessary and to reject that discourse is potentially risky for the patient. But, there remains the possibility of working alongside the medical and identifying spaces of personal reflection and experiential subjectivity, where the gaze can be recuperated, to some extent. In other instances, performance is considered as the site of potentiality in terms of turning the 'vision machine' into something less violent, less judgemental and more humane. Bodies can be staged in ways that draw attention to the potentially brutalizing effects of treating subjects as specimens and it can establish a dynamics of care and an ethics of spectatorship that runs against the persistence of objectifying medical vision and intrusive revelation.

At particular historical moments then, it can be argued that medicine and performance more explicitly intersect. This inevitably occurs when the body is staged as a medical spectacle and it haunts the painful history of human zoos and freak shows through the nineteenth and early twentieth centuries, when 'professionalized medicine consolidated its dominance, casting as pathological all departures from the standard body' (Garland-Thomson, 2008, 60). This moment overlaps with the emergence of naturalism in the theatre, when the theatre itself became the location for experimenting with scientific ideas, as explored in

Shepherd-Barr's essay in this collection. As Darwinian theories of evolution ignited scientists and the public imagination, so the theatre, through Zola, Strindberg, Ibsen and others, became the site for staging and interrogating some of these debates (e.g. Shepherd-Barr, 2015 and 2006; Goodall, 2002). These newly explicit connections between medicine and performance have remained throughout the twentieth century but, as Shepherd-Barr contends, there has been a definite 'surge' of theatrical work interested in science, including medicine, since the mid-1990s and this has 'created a true phenomenon' (2006, 1). So, what might be the impetus for this phenomenon?

Medicine in culture

Health and medicine are now pervasive elements of our cultural discourse, with some 'powerful…icon[s]' in circulation, which impact on our social imaginary and determine how we, the public, engage with particular aspects of medico-science (Anker and Nelkin, 2004, 1). For instance, in relation to genetics, the image of the 'double helix stands in for the gene; it has come to have a ubiquitous presence in contemporary culture as the sign of vitality, immortality, and the future' (Stacey, 2010, 5). Core aspects of our daily existence are now constantly debated, measured, tested and evaluated in relation to our health and well-being, with an eye on 'felt illness' but also future risk, as we encounter the 'public-health logic of awareness' which identifies us all as 'patient[s]-in-waiting' (Dumit, 2012, 56). Part of this cultural landscape has emerged from the 'biologization' of medicine (and many other fields) during the twentieth century. As Lennard J. Davis explains, '[m]ore and more we do see formerly social-political issues, such as race, gender, sexual identity and identity in general, subsumed under the scientific/ medical discourses of genetics, biochemistry, prescription drugs, social and public policy' (2009, online). The suffix 'bio' now shapes a diverse range of disciplines and philosophies, including biomedicine, biotechnology, biopolitics and bioethics. So extensive is this shift that in their *Biocultures Manifesto*, Davis and Morris, propose that 'culture and history must be rethought with an understanding of their inextricable, if highly variable, relation to biology' (2009, online). As the 'bio' has permeated every aspect of the social and the academic, so Davis and Morris outline a necessarily interdisciplinary approach where the humanities and the sciences work together 'to inform and be informed by each other' (2009, online).

Some of this interdisciplinary work is, of course, already underway and has been for some time, in a variety of contexts. For instance, the art exhibition *Spectacular Bodies* at the Hayward Gallery, London, in 2000, and the touring anatomy show, *Bodyworlds*, which first came to the UK in 2002, both engaged with the display and aestheticization of the medicalized human body. There has been a turn, for example, towards an artistic engagement with medical museums, archives and collections, particularly in relation to disability, representation and (in)visibility in these institutions. For instance, Mat Fraser's *Cabinet of Curiosities: How disability was kept in a box*, in 2014, explored the archives of the Science Museum, the Royal College of Physicians and the Hunterian Museum, London, to consider past representations of disability and how museums could be more inclusive in the future. In the UK, a substantial proportion of such work across art, performance and medicine is being enabled by the Wellcome Trust, a charitable foundation that has a particular strand of funding dedicated to exploring 'medicine in culture'. Its aim is to 'embed biomedical science in the historical and cultural landscape, so that it is valued and there is mutual trust between researchers and the wider public' (Wellcome Trust, online). Artists and scholars can access funding through the Wellcome's grant programmes for either public engagement projects or the medical humanities, and such awards have supported a number of the projects explored in this book. Other institutions, such as Arts Catalyst, have also been instrumental in actively promoting and supporting science-art collaborations since the 1990s (see Ede, 2000). This emergence and subsequent flourishing of 'sci-art' projects has continued to the present day, as various organizations and foundations continue to promote science in and through art.

Performance and medicine

Until recently, performance has constituted a relatively minor area of sci-art: visual and film-based projects tend to dominate in much of the literature that deals with this area (e.g. Arends and Thackara,

1999; Ede, 2010; Wilson, 2012; Miller, 2014). However, the late twentieth century marks the emergence of theatre as a growing area of science-arts practice, with the astounding success of Michael Frayn's *Copenhagen* (1998) representing an important milestone in the popularization of this genre. Theatre, dance and live art that engage with medicine or medical sciences represent a particularly vibrant sub-genre of science-engaged performance, with critically acclaimed productions such as Complicite's *Mnemonic* (1999) and, more recently, Headlong Theatre's production of Lucy Prebble's *The Effect* (2012), testifying to its popularity.

However, interdisciplinary engagements between performance and medicine are not confined to theatre plays about biomedical subjects (for instance, the neuroscience of memory formation for *Mnemonic* or effects of mood-altering drugs in *The Effect*). As this volume constitutes one of the few critical responses to this emerging area, we here offer a brief mapping of the various ways in which performance practice and medicine intersect in the contemporary moment. The categories outlined below are distinguished by their aesthetic and ideological orientations, but should not be considered as definitive (particular examples of practice might straddle two or more categories). Moreover, the map should not be considered comprehensive. A broader definition of performance would include other public practices. Indeed, the reader will find that 'performance' is defined more widely in many of the chapters that make up this volume, with discussions encompassing a TEDMed lecture, a pub quiz, hospital-based and gallery installations, for example, as well as the performance of professional or social roles and of ritualized behaviours. In this, we follow the impetus of the academic discipline of performance studies, which extends the purview of drama scholars to consider 'actions' or 'what people do in their activity of doing it' as performance (Schechner, 2013, 1). For now, though, our attention is on performance defined more narrowly, yet still encompassing a range of artistic practices.

The medical in theatre plays

Shepherd-Barr's *Science on Stage* (2006) (a comprehensive mapping of the genre of 'science plays') points to a long 'tradition of depicting the medical profession on stage' that includes canonical works such as Ben Jonson's *The Alchemist* (1610), Ibsen's *An Enemy of the People* (1882) and George Bernard Shaw's *The Doctor's Dilemma* (1906) (2006, 155). Shepherd-Barr suggests that this tradition continues to the present day with numerous examples of 'deft', 'powerful', 'moving and visceral' plays (180) that explore the experiences of doctor and/or patients, including Peter Brook and Marie-Helene Estienne's *The Man Who* (1993), Brian Friel's *Molly Sweeney* (1994) and Margaret Edson's *Wit* (1995). The popularity of these theatrical medical plays lies partly in their engagement with the richly ambivalent status that medicine and the medical profession holds in the popular imagination, and our fascination with the sorts of extraordinary insights that those with serious illness, disability or atypical perception or cognition can convey, and with the drama inherent in the sort of life-changing or life-threatening situations that necessitate medical intervention.

Shepherd-Barr identifies a newer development within the tradition of medical plays: 'plays built on interviews with patients', such as Anna Deavere Smith's untitled work for Yale Medical School (2000), Nell Dunn's *Cancer Tales* (2002) and Mick Gordon's *On Death* (1999). A similar desire for 'true' stories is also reflected in autobiographical work by artists concerning their own experiences of illness e.g. breast-cancer survivor, Linda Park-Fuller, *A Clean Breast of It* (1993) or of disability, for example in Mat Fraser's various works. This rich area of practice forms the subject of Part II of this volume, where live artist and cancer survivor Brian Lobel features as one example of such autobiographical performance.

'Alternative' science plays and the medical

In the last chapter of *Science on Stage*, Shepherd-Barr draws attention to the 'alternative' science play that is characterized by its direct presentation of complex science, rather than mediating this through character and plot (200). In such performances, scientific concepts inspire abstract, experimental forms that engage their audiences experientially rather than intellectually or emotively. We might include in this category contemporary dance or inter-medial performances in which scientific concepts or data provide a choreographic score. It tends to be the 'harder' sciences that are employed in these ways but 'alternative' medical science performances, though few, are significant because they can sometimes represent a different interdisciplinary dynamic to the previous category. The more conventional medical play can serve a 'public engagement' agenda, using drama's ability to provoke emotional engagement to raise interest in medical science and its social impacts: theatre at the service of science. In the 'alternative' form, science can serve as an inspiration for innovative theatrical forms.

Medical performances

'Medical performances' are here defined by their employment of medical procedures and technologies, often enacted upon the artists' body or the use of biological material in the making of living artworks. Artists whose work exemplifies the former include Stelarc, Mona Hatoum, and, two artists whose work features in this volume, Bob Flanagan and Martin O'Brien. Our key example of the latter is Helen Pynor whose chapter in Part III offers an insight into a performance that employs technologies and procedures associated with heart transplant. An important promoter of such 'bio-art' is SymbioticA, a research laboratory based at the University of Western Australia that enables 'artists and researchers to engage in wet biology practices in a biological science department' (website). The work of performance artist, ORLAN, bridges these two forms of 'medical performance': in *The Reincarnation of Saint Orlan* (1990–1993), ORLAN underwent a series of cosmetic surgeries, offering the surgeries themselves, and the presentation of her changing body, as performances. In her more recent project, *Harlequin Coat* (2007), ORLAN used in-vitro culturing technologies to create a garment composed of different people's skin cells. Such works can be seen as a contemporary manifestation of 'body art', a movement emerging out of gallery-based, visual arts practices in the mid-twentieth century, which situated the body as both the object/material of artistic practice, and its subject (see Jones, 1998; O'Reilly, 2009; Jones and Warr, 2012).

In its use of medical procedures and techniques for artistic purposes, this category represents a closer alignment of medicine and performance than other categories. Indeed, a number of its practitioners have specialist medical training (or are, indeed, medical practitioners, for example, Ive Tabar, discussed in Krpic, 2014). This 'complementary' dynamic is similar to that of the following category – despite often very different aesthetic styles.

Theatre-in-health and dramatherapy

Emma Brodzinki's *Theatre in Health and Care* delineates an important 'developing field' of 'medicine, health and care and the performing arts' (2010, 2), which recognizes the capacity of theatre and performance practices to 'promote well-being through engagement in artistic activities' (7), a capacity that has been somewhat undervalued to date, at least in accounts of arts in health (20). Practices discussed in Brodzinski's book 'promote well-being' in different ways – through performances in hospitals, in public health campaigns or the use of actors as simulated patients in medical training, for example. A significant branch of such work seeks to 'give a voice' to those who feel themselves to be socially marginalized by their experiences of chronic illness or disability (see Kuppers, 2014). A related area (though one not discussed in Brodzinski's book) is that of dramatherapy, 'a method of therapy which uses the dramatic process to help people during times of stress, emotional upheaval or disability' (Langley, 2006, 1; see also Jennings, 1997) and that, like theatre-in-health, is defined by its intention to benefit, in this case through psychotherapeutic methodologies. In both these practices, performance shares with medicine a therapeutic intent: performance as a form of medicine. Growing recognition of 'affect' – the embodied emotional and cognitive response of the audience member or participant to an artwork – as the trigger for potential beneficial change (Thompson, 2009) makes this analogy yet more apt. All the more so now that cognitive science urges us to conceptualize audience/participant experiences (that might once have been deemed somewhat nebulous and unquantifiable) in biological terms (McConachie and Hart, 2006; McConachie, 2008 and 2012).

In this overarching therapeutic aim, both theatre-in-health and, more tentatively, dramatherapy can be considered sub-genres of applied theatre, that is, 'forms of dramatic activity that are specifically intended to benefit individuals, communities and societies' (Nicholson, 2014, 3; see also Shaughnessy, 2012). Recent scholarship in this field challenges a distinction that tends to be made by both practitioners and scholars, between applied and purportedly 'aesthetic' theatre (see Jackson, 2007, Shaughnessy, 2012; White, 2015). Because of scholarly discussions emerging elsewhere, we have not dedicated space in this volume to theatre-in-health and dramatherapy, but we strongly endorse these scholars' belief in the potential therapeutic power of all performance practice.

Performance and the medical body

As this suggests, the intersection of performance and medicine in the contemporary moment constitutes a broad and diverse area, and a more comprehensive mapping of the field is beyond the scope of this volume. Our focus is therefore directed upon a single theme that allows us to draw from across this range of practice: the ways in which the body is understood, displayed and represented in performance. We derive the term 'the medical body' from Jennifer Parker-Starbuck's book *Cyborg Theatre* (2014) where it represents a particular instance of the way in which technology and bodies interact on stage and in the social realm. She meditates further on the concept of 'the medical body' in her contribution to this volume: 'If medicine is commonly understood as something applied to a body – a treatment, diagnosis, agent, corrective – then the medical body is one that is acted upon' (Chapter 1). The 'medical body' is one that is 'acted upon' by illness or disability and/or by the diagnostic and therapeutic activities of the medical profession. As such, the medical body – like other cyborg bodies discussed by Parker-Starbuck (2014) – can be both 'abject' (because of their disturbance of normative corporeal organization and control) and rendered into an 'object' (in its passivity to medical intervention). For these medical bodies, subjectivity and agency are effaced by their status as an anatomical object, whether this is as part of a medical procedure (such as transplantation, reproductive technologies or diagnostic analysis) or as a teaching tool, in both formal and informal settings (such as a museum object or a microscope slide). However, the 'medical body' is also a 'subject' (as Parker-Starbuck argues in relation to cyborg bodies), that is, an individual with will and desire. Performance often enables such bodies to enact, act out, up or against the passivity that is often ascribed to the role of the patient or the authority ascribed to the medical professional. In this case, the body is seen as continuous with consciousness, subjectivity, agency, personhood and individuality – and performance is deployed as a practice and a concept that draws attention to these aspects. Sections of this volume single out the 'patient' and the 'specimen' as particular instances of the medical body (as explained below). However, it is important to recognize that the ubiquity of medical practice in contemporary Western society means that to a certain extent we are all 'medical bodies'. The tension highlighted here, between the body as subject and object is familiar to us all.

While this book is concerned with performance and the medical body from the late twentieth century on, its structure parallels the historical development of modern medicine in terms of replicating the move from examining the outside of the body, in holistic terms, to examining its internal and microscopic structures. The sections mirror a medicalized approach, starting with a consideration of the whole body and thinking about a variety of theoretical approaches to the idea of the 'medical body' in performance; the second part examines specific bodies as patients in performance and how their stories are conveyed; and the final section focuses the interrogation still further by exploring anatomized, microscopic and cellular representations. Moving from the macro to the micro, the book echoes the trajectory of the medical gaze and medical practice, and concludes by thinking about cutting edge biomedical-technologies, pointing towards the future.

Part I: Performing the medical

This section frames the medical body in performance by providing some examples of the approaches that might be employed in its study and analysis. In asking how performance and medicine intersect, the chapters here offer insight into the variety of ways that this interface can be explored: through thinking about the way that medical devices and ideas appear in contemporary performance, through its histories, through performative experiences and through the eyes and work of the surgeon. Our medicalized approach is exemplified in these chapters, where different scholars (two of whom are also practitioners) read their cultural and subjective landscapes in relation to a broad understanding of 'medical theatre', which might have 'its own definitions of performance, symptoms, reading practices and audience relations' (Kuppers, 2003, 38). Parker-Starbuck opens this section by using the metaphor of the 'cabinet of curiosities' to collect and identify specific moments of the medical body (and its trace) in contemporary performance. In using the cabinet as a kind of memory machine, Parker-Starbuck reminds us of the ubiquity of medicine in performance and, by extension, within our wider social and political context. The collection in this cabinet of curiosities juxtaposes a range of performance experiences and exposes the relational dynamics at play when we associate artefacts and ideas with each other, such as medicine and performance. The objects in the cabinet (and the essays incorporated here) 'find their meaning only side by side with others, between the walls of a room in which the scholar could measure at every moment the boundaries of the universe' (Agamben, 1994, 30).

Offering a historical approach in the following chapter, Shepherd-Barr traces the 'development of the diagnostic gaze through various examples of the cross-fertilization of medicine and theatre throughout the nineteenth century' (Chapter 2). These intersections take in stagings of the 'freak' body and its legitimizing by medical and scientific practice at the time; the metaphor of dissection in the emergence of theatrical naturalism as a means of undertaking close observation of the subject; and the dramatic presentation of doctors (and some nurses) on the stage. Shepherd-Barr argues that these instances reveal a healthy concern with the increasing dominance and power of doctors and that this legacy, of questioning medicine through theatrical means, remains within contemporary practice.

Kuppers then provides a travelogue of healing spaces, taking the author from New Zealand and a botanical preservation project in the aftermath of the earthquakes in 2010 and 2011, to a sound bath in the deserts of California and back to New Zealand to a hot, natural spa. In adopting Walter Benjamin's figure and practice of the flâneur, Kuppers excavates a range of sites and subjective experiences, where she can be a globalized health tourist and which ends with an invite to the reader to consider their own 'medical adventures' and 'healing tourist anecdotes' (Chapter 3). The section closes with a contribution from Roger Kneebone, and a move to the idea of 'performing surgery'. As a general and trauma surgeon for ten years, then a G.P. and now Professor of Surgical Education at Imperial College, London, Kneebone is pioneering the use of simulated surgical environments as a means of educating the public about the world inside the operating theatre. His work explores the performative aspects of the surgical journey for the patient and the medical team and addresses how performance might be utilized to inform and enhance surgical practice (Chapter 4).

Part II: Performing patients

Part II of this volume is framed by what Emma Brodzinski calls 'embodied pathography' (Chapter 5). Her essay on the 'Patient Performer' stakes out this area of performance practice, which is situated in the overlap between autobiographical performance (see Heddon, 2007) and the literary genre of pathography, that is, personal narratives of illness (see Frank, 1995; Hunsaker Hawkins, 1999). Arthur W. Frank's famous *The Wounded Storyteller* emphasizes that illness narratives are not just 'stories about the body' but also 'stories as told through the body' (1995, 2). However, with embodied pathographies, stories are also told *by* the body: the appearance and actions of these bodies convey 'stories' that might enhance, undercut or replace the spoken narratives. Brodzinski illustrates some of the strategies employed by 'patient performers' Peggy Shaw (on her experience of stroke), Bob Flannagan (whose work explores his life with cystic fibrosis) and Brian Lobel (drawing on his encounter with testicular cancer).

Recognizing the importance of attending to the patient's voice in such practices, we invited one of the artists discussed by Brodzinki to contribute an essay to this volume. Lobel's own chapter in our collection discusses his more recent project with the Birmingham Teenage Cancer Trust, *Fun with Cancer Patients*. Placing these two chapters alongside each other draws out a line of discussion that reveals how embodied pathographies can cut across social constructions of illness or disability. As Sontag famously argued, illness has a metaphorical dimension whereby particular, and often unrealistic, attributes are imposed upon or expected of, those affected: the romantic qualities ascribed to tuberculosis in the nineteenth century or the way in which AIDS is characterized as a biblical plague in the 1980s (2002). In the contemporary moment, cancer is particularly ripe for such metaphorical construction, with a set of behavioural (Ehrenreich, 2009) and narrative (Stacey, 1997) expectations imposed upon those affected by this 'emperor of all maladies' (Mukherjee, 2011b).

Lennox and Pettit's chapter, 'DOC: the narrative performance of expertise' draws attention to the way in which pathographic narratives – in this case circulated by the diabetes online community – can offer alternatives to medical discourses that reduce the patient to a set of symptoms and measurements. In their case study of diabetes blogger Kerri Sparling, they discuss how she uses vlog performances to assert her independence from the 'numbers', the continuous monitoring of her blood sugar and its tacit associations of guilt ascribed to their patterns. However, as Lennox and Pettit argue, such performances also demonstrate a compliance with the operations of the medical profession, as demonstrated in her videos created to endorse medical products. This negotiation of the medical gaze reflects an ambivalent relationship between cultural and medical practices. Part II concludes with a chapter from performance artist Martin O'Brien whose work, like that of Bob Flanagan (discussed by Brodzinski in Chapter 5), engages with the psychosocial experience of living with cystic fibrosis. Both these artists' work foregrounds the body, rather than the spoken word, as a means of opening up 'a discursive space for the exploration of fears and fantasies and alternative ways of being with illness' (Brodzinski). O'Brien's chapter meditates on the cough – as a symptom of cystic fibrosis and an involuntary action that seems to cause disease to those who hear it. In relation to his show, *Regimes of Hardness*, O'Brien asks 'what is at stake when the cough *is* the performance, rather than an introduction to, or interruption of it?' (Chapter 8). In citing Appelbaum's description of the cough as the 'detonation of the voice', we are reminded that embodied pathographies communicate beyond words.

Part III: Performing body parts

In staging bodies or bits of bodies that are objectified, isolated and even examined at the level of the microscopic and cellular, the essays in our final section encounter medical concepts, technologies and its futures as they map onto questions of identity and spectatorial relations. The first two essays are focused on the work of London-based theatre company, Clod Ensemble. Bouchard offers an academic analysis of their piece *Under Glass* by engaging a particular medical concept and then using it to think through and about the performance. It reflects on the work seen, after the bodies have left the stage, whilst Willson's chapter, which follows, dissects the research and the structure of a work as it comes into being. Told from Willson's perspective as an artistic director of Clod Ensemble, she outlines the ideas that informed *An Anatomie in Four Quarters*, and interweaves this with a record of the arrangement and central actions of the performance. Part rehearsal notes, part performance archive, part philosophical reflection, this essay writes the body and its moves as it emerges on stage for a finished production. These two different voices and approaches write the medical body in performance in different but mutually productive ways.

In more detail, Bouchard's essay examines the medical concept of 'specimens' in relation to Clod Ensemble's work *Under Glass* (2010). By utilizing a scientific and medical idea of creating specimens for research and in thinking about how the specimen is constructed and made to perform its function through isolation and display, Bouchard considers how performance can avoid some of medicine's brutalizing features and establish more ethical spectatorial dynamics. Indeed, her argument that *Under Glass* draws us back to an 'ethics of care and responsibility for those identified as specimens' frames the subsequent chapters (Chapter 9). It also articulates a key premise of the volume as a whole: the capacity of performance to evoke empathetic, and, through this, an ethical engagement with the 'medical body'. The focus then remains with Clod Ensemble, as Suzy Willson's chapter provides rehearsal notes and research for her work from 2011, with Clod Ensemble, *An Anatomie in Four Quarters*, first staged at Sadler's Wells, London. The piece deliberately explores the 'vision machine' of anatomy and dance theatre, through closely associating theatre and historical practices of anatomical dissection in its creation. These impacted on the form and the structure of the piece, which both anatomized the theatre architecture, at the same time as dissecting the histories of anatomy and movement. Willson's contribution provides a unique archive of the work's interface with medicine and its histories (Chapter 10).

There follows another practitioner's contribution, as visual artist Helen Pynor writes about her installation and performance work, *The Body is a Big Place*, which was created over the period 2010–2013 (Chapter 11). It engaged with organ transplantation and 're-enacted' some aspects of the human heart transplant process. The piece involved the perfusion of a pair of pig hearts alongside a video installation of members of an Australian organ transplant community. The essay incorporates different voices and narratives about death, and signals the liminal space between life and death, organ transplantation and her experience of making the work. Like Willson's contribution, this 'essay' is written in a quite different mode from the more academic pieces included in the volume. Drawing on a range of sources that are a mixture of the medical and the poetic, the piece interweaves research for the piece with Pynor's own working notes and the reader encounters a strong sense of different voices, imperatives and tones in the writing, as they are gathered together in one place. What comes across particularly strongly in Pynor's writing is the sense of highly specific and technical language around medical knowledge and practice, which is underpinned by advanced technologies. These technologies mediate between bodies in these instances, making the transplant from one body to another possible, for example. These final chapters depend on an explicit engagement with such biotechnologies, as they turn towards the level of the cellular and the microscopic and issues of what to represent and how to represent the medical body become more pressing. Mermikides provides insight into the difficulties of performing 'microscopic anatomies' in a variety of contexts and examples. As van Dijck argues: 'Imaging technologies claim to make the body transparent, yet their ubiquitous use renders the interior body more technologically complex. The more we see through various camera lenses, the more complicated the visual information becomes … the mediated body is everything but transparent; it is precisely this complexity and stratification that makes it a contested cultural object' (van Dijick, 2005, 4). For the performance maker, the question of how to make the cellular meaningful and legible to an audience becomes key and Mermikides considers the strengths and pitfalls of some of this work (Chapter 12).

The final essay in the book likewise deals with cutting edge medical and scientific advances, as we journey towards what might be on our biomedical horizon of regenerative medicine and synthetic biology. Gabriella Giannachi explores the work of media artist Lynn Hershman Leeson and her current piece *The Infinity Engine*. The piece is staged in a replica genetics lab and the audience are spectators of and participants in experimental biomedical work. In response to this work, which is part performance, part science laboratory, part archive, part experiment, Giannachi proposes a new 'organic performance framework', which moves beyond Hassan's familiar modernist/post-modernist dichotomy. This organic performance framework reflects on the nature of the work as both art and science, as a product in and of itself, yet that is also generative. For Giannachi, we are still experiencing the post-modern 'condition' but we have moved to an engagement with the body and, more specifically the medical body, as one that is potentially being regenerated from the inside out, and as such this requires a new framework for analysis and critical thought. The proposition of a new means of evaluating such work suggests the kinds of theoretical models we might develop and deploy in relation to the interface between performance and medicine, in all its complexity. As such, it offers a platform for future scholarship that might extend the discussions, opened in this volume, on the interdisciplinary overlap between performance and science.

Interdisciplinary dialogues

As this book launches a series of 'interdisciplinary dialogues', it is worth dwelling here on the concept of interdisciplinarity as it is represented within its pages. Shaughnessy's introduction to *Cognitive Science and Affective Performance* (2013, the inspiration for this series), argues for the value of 'thinking in threes', rather than in binaries in the context of interdisciplinary endeavours. It is for this reason that our volume is not strictly or straightforwardly a two-way dialogue between the disciplines of performance and medicine, but also engages with the body. In this, we follow the recuperation, within arts practices, of the body as 'a credible subject and medium' (O'Reilly, 7) and 'a veritable explosion of interest' in the body (Fraser and Grecos, 2005, 1) as the focus of interdisciplinary analysis (e.g. van Dijck, 2005; Sheets-Johnstone, 2009; Lupton, 2012).

The body thereby provides a bridge between performance and medicine. In situating itself in the overlaps between these domains, our project pertains to the evolving field of medical humanities, which brings together scholars and professionals situated in both medical and humanities departments, and employs theoretical frameworks from a diverse range of disciplines alongside medicine, such as history, sociology, cultural studies, arts and literary studies[1] (e.g. Evans and Finlay, 2001; Bates and Bleakley, 2013; Cole et al., 2014; Bates et al. 2015). Indeed, a key aim of this collection is to bolster the increasing recognition of performance within medical humanities. Until very recently, the study of the arts in the medical humanities has tended to neglect performance practices. An example of this is Cole, Carlin and Carlson's textbook, which contains chapters on literature, poetry, film and media but none on theatre, dance or performance. A welcome exception is Bates, Bleakley and Goodman's *Medicine, Health and the Arts* (2015), which includes a section on performance.

The 'interdisciplinary dialogue' encompassed within these pages cannot be construed simply as one between 'art' and 'science'. For the clinical practice of medicine, which is the main concern of most of our contributors, is commonly regarded as an applied science, with only laboratory-based research claiming the title of 'pure' science. Indeed, it has been argued that clinical practice is as much an art as it is a science (e.g. Malterud, 2001; Petros, 2001). Likewise, as both an artform and an academic discipline,[2] performance is disciplinarily promiscuous, regularly bringing into dialogue a set of constitutive and aligned arts (music, design, dance, visual arts, digital technologies and so on), and engaging with humanities subjects (such as history and political theories), and some 'softer' scientific disciplines (e.g. sociology, psychology, human anatomy and increasingly, cognitive science).

The disciplinary promiscuity of performance as an artform is especially evident in two of the chapters that are written by artists, Suzy Willson (Chapter 10) and Helen Pynor (Chapter 11). Each of these collates an impressive range of sources and voices from distinct areas of practice that inspired the projects under discussion: historical concepts of anatomy and medical art in Willson's account of *Anatomie in Four Quarters*; the blending of professional, technical and personal voices in Pynor's reflections upon *The Body is a Big Place*. These chapters are also examples of 'performative writing', a radicalization of conventional academic writing that allows for the contingency of knowledge (often by placing contradictory texts in relation to each other) and, in keeping with its routes in feminism, the inclusion of the personal within its pages (see Phelan, 1997, 11–12). Thus, again, we see how the broad definition of performance that underpins this volume can expand the possibilities inherent in particular disciplines (in this case the academy) and render more porous the borders between them (such as those that distinguish the arts and the academy).

The array of disciplines represented by our contributors already share common languages and concerns, yet there is much to be gained through discussions such as those contained in this book. The volume, then, might be the best thought of as the sort of dialogue that occurs at a party – among friends old and new, friends of friends and strangers – rather than in a formal interview. Some conversations build on shared history and knowledge, revealing new points of conflict and commonality; others are the start of a longer discussion. All, we hope, will lead to further dialogue for, ultimately, this book acts as both an introduction and a provocation to future work in an exciting and growing area of interdisciplinary debate.

PART ONE

Performing the Medical

1

A Cabinet of (Medical) Performance Curiosities

Jennifer Parker-Starbuck

I've got time to give just one of you a gut reading with this portable ultrasound device, so is there anyone here who would like a gut reading? Great. I'm just going to ask you to apply this bit of gel. It's a bit cold, sorry. Now just hold this over your stomach and press [...] Hang on, I'm getting an image. It's a bit grainy but bear with it ... can you see?

(HILL AND PARIS, 2014, 70)

Imagine, if you will, an immense cabinet, perhaps made of ornately carved and oiled wood, full of shelves and drawers and nooks and crannies separated by panes of glass, within which hundreds of curiosities can be found. Now imagine this cabinet full of the images, bodies and moments that occur to you when you think of 'the medical body in performance'. What sorts of things would fill these spaces? This chapter took shape as I imagined just this, a literal 'Cabinet of Curiosity' filled with the 'medical bodies' of my own performance experiences. I fixed upon the portable ultrasound device (described above) used in Curious' (Leslie Hill and Helen Paris) *the moment i saw you i knew i could love you*

(2009 ongoing), I imagined the medical chair used in The Wooster Group's *To You, The Birdie!* (2001–2006), I recalled the leg brace dancer Cathy Weis wore in her piece *Not So Fast, Kid* (2001), I pondered the cyborg bodies transformed by technologies, at the service of medical or scientific experimentation, that prompted my metaphoric use of the cyborg in my book *Cyborg Theatre* (2011). In this chapter I construct and offer a Cabinet of (medical) Curiosities that explores not only bodies but also memories, body parts and augmentations. It is inspired by the historical development of these cabinets including, for example, the seventeenth-century collection of Francisco Calzolari in Italy and the 'ark' collection inherited by Elias Ashmole later in the same century (which became the Ashmolean Museum, Oxford), and contemporary museum 'cabinets', such as the Mütter Museum in Philadelphia or the Hunterian Museum in London, in which objects have been curated to perform a kind of 'wonder', a history brought together over time and place. The Cabinet of Curiosity is a metaphor for dualities, as Patrick Mauriès describes: 'their intention was not merely to define, discover and possess the rare and the unique, but also, and at the same time, to inscribe them within a special setting which would instil in them layers of meaning' (2002, 25). As I thought more about my imagined 'cabinet', images and moments within my performance history began to fill the spaces, sitting in awkward juxtapositions, reminding me of the frailty and strength of the (medical) body.

But what is a 'medical body'? Is it a body displayed, cut open, or operated on? Is it an ill body, a traumatized body, a psychologically damaged body? Is this body physically riddled with pain or disease? Is it a cyborg body, such as the first cyborg rat, a white lab rat fitted with an osmotic pump on its tail, used to research conditions for human space travel? This modified laboratory animal symbolizes a starting point for my thinking about many types of medically augmented bodies. If medicine is commonly understood as something applied to a body – a treatment, diagnosis, agent, corrective – then the medical body is the one that is 'acted upon'. Like cyborg bodies, reliant on external hands to conjoin or implant the non-organic element in the living flesh, medical bodies are ripe with internal and external tensions, and represent the blurring of dualities such as life/death, animate/ inanimate and public/private.

Shelf 1: Stelarc's *Stomach Sculpture*. My Cabinet of (Medical) Curiosity would not be complete without an entry from Australian performance artist Stelarc. Well known for his living sculptures of 'the body' (his preferred term for his own body) hanging from hooks over various locations in the 1980s, it is his *Stomach Sculpture* that poses questions for me about the medical body in performance. In the piece, executed in 1993, he inserts a specially constructed sculpture attached to a camera, into his stomach. The procedure is a medical one and he had difficulty finding a doctor to assist him. He explains that 'The stomach sculpture is actually the most dangerous performance I've done. We had to be within 5 minutes of a hospital in case we ruptured any internal organs' (Stelarc, 1995). Stelarc describes the process:

> To insert the sculpture...the closed capsule, with beeping sound and flashing light activated, was swallowed and guided down tethered to it's [sic] flexidrive cable attached to the control box outside the body. Once inserted into the stomach, we used an endoscope to inflate the stomach and suck out the excess body fluids. The sculpture was then arrayed with switches on the control box. We documented the whole performance using video endoscopy equipment. (Stelarc, 1995)

Stelarc's stomach sculpture blurs the lines between a medical procedure and performance, between inside and outside. He turns his performing body into a medical body, but offers viewers a chance to perform a medical gaze, often restricted to medical doctors. Although difficult to 'swallow', the piece makes the private world public, perhaps assuaging some of the anxiety over this kind of procedure.

The 'medical bodies' that form the basis of this chapter are representative of the complexity of these dualities, and they are framed within this imaginary Cabinet of Curiosity as, in some way, cyborgean, that is, constructed through the understanding of bodies that are 'acted upon'. When I take the ultrasound equipment and 'apply the gel' and press down, my grainy images of the medical body in performance are not only the bodies themselves but also the prostheses, props, fragments, objects, tools, instruments and machines that augment the bodies and that shift corporeal borders into the medical. Like Cabinets of old, also known as *Wunderkammer*, or Chambers of Wonders, these examples might provide an antidote, or performative 'care' when faced with medical narratives in our own lives. As Christine Davenne points out in *Cabinets of Wonder*, 'the term "curiosity" itself derives from the Latin *cura*: "which takes care"', and the cabinets were full of potential pharmaceuticals: 'Princes acquired countless viper tongues, unicorn horns (actually narwhal horns), rhinoceros horns, toad skins and skulls, and bezoars, which they carefully stored in a specific furniture piece in their cabinet called the "pharmacy"' (2011, 133). This medical Cabinet of Curiosity gathers together brief examples, some more obvious than others, of 'medical bodies' in my performance imagination. This essay is designed as a curated cabinet of shelves and drawers full of reflection and connection between performance and medicine.

Shelf 2: The 'Wooster Group chair': Somewhere in the centre of my cabinet sits what I call the 'Wooster Group chair'. Although a version has been used in many productions, the chair is most memorable to me from the Wooster Group's *To You, the Birdie!*, an exploration of, among other things, Racine's *Phèdra*. The chair becomes a physicalized extension of Kate Valk's silent Phèdre and is a potent symbol of her suffering and incapacity to act as Queen. The chair, a medical shower chair on wheels, is made of aluminium poles and a toilet seat, and for this production was attached to an IV pole with an enema bag hooked on top. It seemed to trail Valk around the stage, ready, alongside her Nurse Oenone, to be of assistance. The 'Wooster Group chair' may not have been intended to resonate so with a medical world of tubes and indignities – several were originally purchased for *Brace Up!* for their manoeuvrability. Liz LeCompte explained to Andrew

Quick in *The Wooster Group Workbook* that she 'found the chairs in a medical catalogue. I was looking for something with very good casters on them. Those particular chairs are shower chairs. They have to be able to be moved into a shower and then turned in a tight circle, so all four casters are movable and all four casters can be locked' (2007, 107). In *Birdie!* however, the chair stands out as a central symbol of a medicalized body, unable to act without assistance, relying on medical equipment for survival. Its intended use as a medical object begins to blur with its performance use and it suddenly reads as medical. It then becomes, through its use in other productions, a 'ghost prop', from its association as the bare display of Phèdre's most private world, to its appearance under cover as Emperor Jones's puppet throne, and then again as a careening throne for the prince Hamlet, who, in their production, himself ghosts the filmed version of Richard Burton's 1964 *Hamlet*, questioning then, now and always, what it means 'to be'? This 'ghosting', as Marvin Carlson would call it, brings with it a sense of a medical body, one perhaps not fully well, not fully agential (Carlson, 2001). The chair then sits on my shelf as a *memento mori*, a reminder of the body's potential frailty, and of a cyborgean reliance on technologies so often associated with medical conditions.

Framing these examples within a Cabinet of Curiosity is not to suggest that these are definitive cases of the medical body, but rather, to look at them as liminal objects, between performance and medicine, between public and private spaces – so often where realities of medical bodies find themselves. Although historically Cabinets of Curiosity have often been foundational items within museums, they began as private collections, microcosms of the much larger, unknown world. Dating back to the sixteenth century, Cabinets of Curiosity describe exotic collections obtained by educated, royal or elite personages to contemplate, and feel in control of, the larger world. They were often rooms full of paintings, objects, specimens or frequently collections of the 'natural' world. The collections represent a historic turn towards a private culture, and, as explained by Davenne: 'By forsaking the collective values embodied by medieval Christianity, the Renaissance introduced a separation between the private and public realms, both in legislation and in monuments... the new area brought knowledge into the intimate spheres of chatting, alcoves, and secrets' (2011, 57). These early collections are symbolic of an attempt to represent a microcosm of the world, but also signify an uncertainty about what exists beyond the boundaries of the known. Although they later become sites for more ordered classification systems that become codified behind the locked display cases of museums, early Cabinets were eclectic, crammed with objects that demanded reflection and connection.

Shelf 3: Dancer Cathy Weis's leg brace. I began researching New York dancer and multimedia artist Cathy Weis because of her innovative uses of technology, TVs, screens, international tele-connected performances (in days pre-Skype). What I learned was that she had turned to media in performance in part due to having multiple sclerosis, which was slowly weakening her right side. Over the years, she began to wear a leg brace when she performed to stabilize her movement and I have vivid memories of her movement sequence in her piece *Not So Fast Kid!*, a production that took place between performers in New York and in Macedonia. She danced with the brace, moving around the space while relating to the projected image of her Macedonian dance partner Robert. Thinking about her movement reminds me of something she said (which I used in my book *Cyborg Theatre* but worth repeating here): 'All movement is interesting – it's how you deal with it. On crutches, or wearing a brace, this movement is as interesting as a ballet dancer's if it has its own voice' (Parker-Starbuck, 2011, 71). On Weis the brace becomes a conduit, helping us to 'hear' this movement differently. It is both an acknowledgement of the medical condition she lives with, but also a symbol of her ability to continue to create new dance. The medical body may be augmented, but it need not be diminished.

In *Cabinets of Curiosities*, Mauriès explains that the cabinets were about 'the knowledge of liminal objects that lay on the margins of charted territory, brought back from worlds unknown, defying any accepted system of classification (and most notably the conventional categories of 'arts' and 'sciences'), and associated with the discovery of 'new worlds' (2002, 12). Like these cabinets, bodies caught up in medical processes resonate with their qualities: shimmering with bits of a life unknown to try to find a sense of order, caught between the private and the public realms, on display, thought about and researched.

Drawer 1: Collections and Collecting

When I think of Cabinets of Curiosity in art and performance practices I think specifically about artist Mark Dion's 1999 piece *Tate Thames Dig* in which he took a team of volunteers to the banks of the Thames, in London, at low tide and collected debris, bones, toys, and whatever they found there.[1] The piece was being developed as the Tate Modern was being finished and was on display as it opened. Like much of Dion's other work, it is a literal Cabinet of Curiosities and the collected objects are arranged and displayed in a large wooden cabinet with drawers of different sizes and display cupboards. I remember being fascinated by the collection, opening and closing the drawers, trying to figure out how they were organized, imagining how these objects got into the Thames and how the water changed their shapes. The collection defied systems of classification, as it merged the past and the present, jumbling items together for the viewer to make sense of.

The histories of Cabinets of Curiosities detail the different modes of collections that filled the cases and spaces of these cabinets (and rooms), from the seemingly chaotic or eclectic personal collections that were used to educate royal family members to those of scientific classification, art, personal trophies, or curated for museums or as the basis of an artwork, and more. Collections, as Susan M. Pearce explains, 'are an important part of our effort to construct the world' (1994, 194). She describes three modes of collecting: 'collections as souvenir', 'fetish objects' and 'systematics' that play out relations between subjects and 'the object, conceived as the whole world, material and otherwise, which lies outside him or her' (1994, 194). The collections themselves, whether souvenirs from selected moments in a life, fetishistic or obsessive collections where accumulation is the goal, or a more systematic approach based on classification, emerge as relational – a blurring of subject and object that might tell us something about a particular moment in history.

Shelf 4: Tim Crouch's *My Arm*. A story about a ten-year-old boy who decided to hold up his arm until it became both a psychological and medical condition has stuck with me since I saw it in New York in 2004. It is this arm, held up above the body throughout a life (and in my mind, throughout the performance, though this is not the case) that I remember so vividly. But also it sticks with me because part of the performance is reliant upon objects gathered from our pockets and handbags which are given to Crouch to perform with for the duration of the show. These inanimate objects take on a life in the performance, animated as icons and memories and people. The notion of the arm as object, the body as object and the incredible powers of control that here created a medical specimen, run through the piece. The boy, who began holding his arm up as a 'game', a form of contest of control against his older brother, takes it too far, and in the fictitious world of the performance he eventually becomes disabled:

> When I was 22 I became officially registered as disabled. Bits of me kept breaking down and then they were fixed. I was in and out of hospitals with various blood infections. My lungs collapsed. I lost weight. At one point a doctor suggested that if I wanted to live a normal life I would have to have my arm amputated...I conceded to having this finger removed. (Crouch, 2011a, np)

The story of this child transforming his body, through sheer determination, into a medical body resonates with stories of self-harm and eating disorders. It reminds me of the tense borders between well and ill, able and dis/abled and while it found a way to connect to my life, its story-telling techniques have a wider application.

This chapter's collection oscillates between Pearce's 'souvenir' and 'systematics'. The examples are personal to me, resonant of my past experiences, and linked to personal medical experiences and conditions. In this sense, they are not comprehensive or systematic case studies intended to speak to any larger audience. Like souvenirs, they, as Pearce explains, 'possess the survival power of materiality not shared by words, actions, sights and the other elements of experience, they alone have the power to carry the past into the present. Souvenirs are samples of events which can be remembered, but not relived' (1994, 195). The examples herein fall into this description as pieces of an experience, freezing and remembering time. With these memories I can grasp an aspect of the performance, they serve as traces of these performances that I take with me. They prepare me, and allow me alternative experiences through which to stage medical journeys.

However, in staging this Cabinet here, in a public space, my collection also cannot help but be, in part, considered as systematic. These kinds of collections, Pearce cautions, appear to stand in for others of their kind, serially, and are displayed as such. They depend upon 'principles of organization which are perceived to have external reality beyond the specific material under consideration, and which are held to derive from general principles deduced from the broad mass of kindred material through the operation of observation and reason' (1994, 201). While some of the examples may well speak to larger questions of how we classify the 'medical' body, or remind readers of their own experiences in medical scenarios, in presenting them here, I am also aware of Pearce's reminder that 'our systematic collections do not show us external reality; they only show us a picture of ourselves' (1994, 202). In this sense then, this chapter is both personal and public, tracing examples that illuminate a kind of thinking about the 'medical body' in performance through a personal account.

Collections are, inevitably, defined and understood by what gets to be included. In Dion's *Tate Thames Dig*, for example, the arrangement of diverse and anachronistic items encourages viewers to think about the histories (items range from teeth from the bear-baiting pits in the Renaissance to mobile phones) and how material culture is sedimented, layered and juxtaposed. The examples I include here are arguably eclectic, and I am not attempting to stake a claim for the most cited or significant examples of medical bodies in performance. If so, I would offer ORLAN's 'Carnal Art'

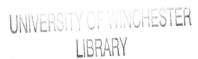

series of body modifications that famously transformed her own face to resemble iconic art works from the *Mona Lisa* to *Venus de Milo*. In an adjacent case might be Ron Athey, whose ongoing extreme body performance explores questions of pain and blood-letting, drawing attention to HIV, which he has lived with since the mid 1980s. Another space would be reserved for Bob Flanagan and Sheree Rose, whose masochistically driven performances were developed to help combat Flanagan's cystic fibrosis. The medical body is not new to performance art. There are many examples to choose from, but in the spirit of the Cabinet of Curiosity I am relying on my own memories, which do range from the obvious to the obscure, as a kind of memory-machine that might assist in processing how to care, how to cope and how to understand the physical challenges and emotional complexities around medical experiences.

Drawer 2: Memory Theatre and Medical Memories

'It is likely that the physical organization of this material Renaissance world picture was dependent on a contemporary cognitive method, the art of memory.' (Hooper Greenhill, 1992, 84)

The examples here attempt to form a bridge between the private and the public. I put the 'items on the shelves' but I leave them with the reader as a snapshot of how different bodies, props and ideas are used in performance to understand and represent both medical themes and our personal connections to what we see. In museum studies, Cabinets of Curiosity have been something of an unknown because of the contents' relationship to the individual collector and it has not always been easy to determine the exact rationale behind a collection. Eileen Hooper Greenhill explains that 'Cabinets of the World' encompassed worlds of libraries and theatres alike. They emerged in relation to who the owner/collectors were – princes, scholars, or merchants – and what financial, intellectual, or political positions of power they held (1992, 102). Placing my memories into a 'Cabinet' hearkens back to the Cabinets as *theatrum mundi*, microcosms of a (my) larger (theatre-going) world. The Cabinet also functions as a kind of memory-theatre, in which a visualization of space solidifies memories. Like the memory-theatre proposed in Guilio Camillo's 1550 *L'Idea del Theatro*, the Cabinet can store traces of these performances to provide 'a physical model for memorization' (Malkin, 1999, 2). Camillo's theatre, based on

Vitruvius's Roman theatre, was structured around the display of images over seven sections on different levels. In her book *Memory-Theatre and Postmodern Drama*, Jeanette Malkin writes that 'Camillo's memory building was devised so that the spectator stood at its center, where the stage should have been, surrounded by the profusion of potent icons. These signs would become meaningful through their relationship with the specific viewer' (1999, 3).

Shelf 5: A water bottle filled with urine. In *Blood* (2013), Jean Abreu's dance-theatre piece, the visual images are full of images of bodily fluids.[2] Inspired by Gilbert and George's 1996 *The Fundamental Pictures*, Abreu asked if he could use them in a performance and they consented.[3] Their saturated close-ups of microscopic cells and bodily fluids – semen, faeces, spit, urine, blood – are projected across the white walls and onto Abreu's white suit. He dances, beautifully, in projected pools of blood as he recites his name, age, height, the condition of his body, indicating, perhaps, a physical check-up, or medical processing. He touches himself as if external hands are upon him. He drinks and spits from a water bottle on stage, he sweats profusely; the piece is filled with many bodily fluids, real and projected. At one point, Abreu, with his back to the audience, urinates into this bottle, and sets it on the floor. Later, he picks it up and dances with it. It isn't often you watch a performer dance a duet with a bottle of their own urine, and it mesmerizes for the rest of the piece. The bottle becomes a physical manifestation of the many bodily fluids represented throughout the piece and this 'sample' seems to be the entry into a medical world where all of these secretions are measured, tested and scrutinized. In the end, the piece leaves me with a feeling that his is a medical body – a body tested, perhaps a body suffering an accident, or a body confronting disease. What remained was this sample, a marker of testing and waiting, of routine and of the unknown.

As I look around my Cabinet, I realize there are many more performances I could fill this space with. I am also acutely aware that each example is also an echo of some of the bodies that have surrounded me; family, friends, loved ones, who have experienced or are experiencing what it means to fall into a category of the medical body. I remember Peggy Shaw's return to the stage post-stroke in her London performance of *RUFF* (April 2013). I saw it not long after my mother's brain surgery and I felt an incredible sense of elation at Shaw's return to the stage.[4] I was also afraid – that she might fall, or forget where she was – but her funny, honest and poignant piece put her body in front of us all, asking for help if she forgot and making us aware of the strength of this act. I also remember being unable to hold back tears as Helen Paris embodied the mixed-up words and objects of a mind forgetting in Curious' latest production, *Best Before End* (May 2013). The piece revolved around a large arm-chair and Paris's poetic and beautiful attempts to push it and lift it and carry it (and its occupier) surrounded me with familiarity as I related to the world of dementia my grandmother had fallen into, never to return. These and many other performances serve as a kind of cure, they make me feel less alone, more aware of the complexities around these conditions. These performances broaden the contours of the medical experience, so often private and unspoken; they ease the symptoms and conditions for others.

Drawer 3: The Medical Unknown

None of us is immune to illness, to aging, to accidents, to disease, to death. Our bodies, if they have not yet been, will become medical bodies at some point. It is inevitable. Yet, when approaching illness it becomes clear how ill-prepared we are to deal with it. Most of us don't understand the terminologies, the science, the treatment options. Most of us don't understand the feeling that comes over us as we try to understand how to be in the world of, affected by, or next to, illness. Worlds change and language shifts. We stand between life and death:

> This dialectic between life and death, this infatuation with the aesthetic transfiguration wrought by death, recurs at an even deeper level, informing the very organization of the collection. It is central, indeed, to the thesis underlying the cabinet of curiosities: for the aim of any collection is to halt the passage of time, to freeze the ineluctable progress of life or history, and to replace it with the fragmented, controllable, circular time frame established by a finite series of objects that can be collected in full. (Mauriès, 2002, 119)

By constructing this Cabinet of (Medical) Performance Curiosities I have begun to collect the medical bodies and objects and moments, perhaps in homeopathic, perhaps in cathartic and perhaps in antidotal ways, that allow me to find a way to understand these worlds differently, through performance.

Shelf 6: The Portable Sonogram Machine

Here comes something … yes, it's faint but it's there – see just there? There is a dark area here. This is very interesting. I think we can all see clearly that this is … land. And it seems to be covered with very fine grey almost like a powder – plaster-of-Paris grey. Let's magnify the image. Now, if you look just here, see these faint impressions? Footprints. From what I can see, this looks like a place where you used to feel very at home, very happy. And even though you haven't been there in a long time, we can see that you are still carrying it inside you. Beautiful. Is that what you expected? Is that what you were hoping for?
(Hill and Paris, 2014, 70–71)

I end as I began, sitting in a large life raft in a cool dark space in the Curious' show, *the moment i saw you i knew i could love you*. This show is a manifestation of research Hill and Paris did into 'gut feelings', what they describe as 'a topography of instinct and impulse, where desire, fear, anger, humiliation or panic occasionally hits us unawares like a rogue wave' (Hill and Paris, 2014, 62). They conducted research for this work at the Wingate Institute of Neurogastroenterology, and the piece is full of scientific images, projections of inner organs or fluids moving through the body. We, the audience, are on a journey, out at sea, into the unknown. During the performance, a performer carries a portable device, small, flat, white and box-shaped, with cord and transducer end attached, and asks to see inside the belly of an audience member. The performer asks the member of the audience if he can rub gel on her belly, before handing her the transducer and having her rub it across her stomach. Here is a medical instrument that can represent joy, sadness or fear depending on the medical scenario. But here, being used in performance, it shifts our attention for a moment, from its medical application to an instrument of the imagination. Through it we look out, into an unknown future, differently. With care, and with hope.

2

The Diagnostic Gaze: Nineteenth-Century Contexts for Medicine and Performance

Kirsten E. Shepherd-Barr

In a special issue of *Modern Drama* in 2008 on theatre and medicine, Stanton B. Garner, Jr noted how surprising it is that little attention has been paid to 'the intersections of theatre and medicine in modern drama' especially since both fields saw great changes and innovations over the late nineteenth and early twentieth centuries: theatre becoming 'modern' and medicine claiming 'new authority' and 'cultural prestige' (2008, 313). Indeed, not only are the roots of the late twentieth-century rise of performance studies firmly grounded in the nineteenth century, they are inextricably linked with a turn towards medicine at the time that was prompted by, on the one hand, increasing specialization within the field of medicine and, on the other hand, increasing authority gained by the medical profession. Both developments are part of the general biocentrism of the period, when advances in science, particularly evolutionary theory, focused attention on the body and taught people to 'gaze' at it in ways that at once anatomized it but also made it an object of spectatorship and performance. George Henry Lewes's observation in 1875 that 'we are all spectators of ourselves' (1875, 103) captures the new spirit of performance saturating Victorian culture, but it tells only part of the story, for it misses out the ways in which we are also all spectators of *each other*, training on our fellow humans a diagnostic gaze shaped by the deepening cultural embeddedness of medical discourse. This chapter traces the development of the diagnostic gaze through various examples of the cross-fertilization of medicine and theatre throughout the nineteenth century.

Freakery

The pairing of theatre with medicine is not surprising. As Garner, Jr. explains, in his definitive discussion of the subject, medical practice 'identifies and pathologizes extra-ordinary bodies in biological terms' and in addition, 'drama, theatre, and performance studies' all deal with 'the body's personal and social performances' (2008, 314). From the Hottentot Venus through bearded women, circus performers and 'freaks', from human anomalies to the commercially displayed peoples or 'ethnological exhibits' popular throughout Europe, the body was on display, a thing of wonder and of constant interplay between the normative and the Other. The showmen who managed the Hottentot Venus, Jocko, bearded women and the like all traded on the growing public appetite for the display of the anomalous human body.[1] Indeed the fascination with freaks encompasses both the living and the dead. This wasn't just voyeurism; 'the printed and physical afterlives of freaks ... became important sites of reference in the development of medical knowledge in the latter part of the Victorian era' (Pettit, 2012, 62). Many of these acts have become powerful cultural memories, revisited over the past century for instance by Arthur Wing Pinero in his 1918 play *The Freaks*, e. e. cummings in his 1946 play *Him*, and more recently in Bernard Pomerance's *The Elephant Man* (1977), Suzan Lori-Parks's *Venus* (1996), Mary Vingoe's *Living Curiosities; or, What You Will* (2011) and Shaun Prendergast's *The True History of the Tragic Life and Triumphant Death of Julia Pastrana, the Ugliest Woman in the World* (1998).[2] This retro-Victorianism shows that not only are we attracted in spite of ourselves to the 'freak' body and its mysterious conditions, but also we feel compelled to reinvent and recast their stories from our own perspective. It's a kind of doubly invasive gaze.

That freak show promoters employed 'medical language' indicates that they were self-consciously situating themselves and their performers within 'a wider practice of popular scientific interactions' (Pettit, 2012, 63). Nineteenth-century performances of medicine are often motivated and characterized by the 'respectable rhetoric of science and medicine' and 'discourses of improvement and novelty' (Kember, Plunkett and Sullivan, 2012, 5). But the revelation of medical mysteries was big business as well as educational, making the medical profession simultaneously aware of how it can engage the public through theatrical techniques and suspicious of the low showmanship with which such spectacle was associated. As Beverley Rogers has shown, doctors were 'uneasily proximate' to freak showmen's practices. Mummy unwrappings went from being 'theatrical stagings' to being at least ostensibly 'educational, investigative events' by the later part of the century, reflecting the tendency for medicine to become less associated with showmanship over the course of the century (Rogers, 2012, 208). It is not surprising that most areas of medicine 'grew less inclined to public display as the century progressed' (Kember, Plunkett and Sullivan, 2012, 8–9). The closed world of medical schools seemed to resist any incursion from performance; lectures could be 'intolerably dull', as Charles Darwin recollected about his training at Edinburgh, with lectures so bad that they were 'fearful to remember' and deeply upsetting visits to the operating theatre at Edinburgh Hospital (in De Beer, 1983, 25–26). This was in the 1820s. The following decades witnessed a flowering of medical performance in the public sphere, the most intense period of their convergence and mutual exchange, before once again moving apart in what Pettit calls 'the separation of medicine from popular entertainment' (2012, 64).

This illustrates the uneven nature of the dynamic between medicine and performance; it is a complex engagement that arguably goes in waves rather than in steady, progressively deeper intertwining. At the core of this shifting relationship is the question of who, in today's terminology, is a stakeholder in such performances. Increased knowledge brings professionalization and specialization, and above all power and authority; these were not to be compromised by association with popular performance, spectacle and theatricality. Indeed, terms like 'spectacle', 'display', and 'show' all emphasize performance as superficial and visual, not something that has to be hunted for but is immediately accessible. While popular performance revolved around this kind of visuality, the discourse of medicine was increasingly about penetration, unwrapping the mysteries of the body through skills that only specialized medical training could allow.

Dissection

At the heart of medical performances touched on so far is the idea of penetration: the revelation of what lies beneath the skin through dissection. This concept is central to both modern medicine and the new movement of naturalistic theatre. Long before being incorporated into mainstream drama through naturalism (and then mainly in a figurative sense, as in playwrights dissecting society through their plays), dissection had been a mainstay of public performance through medical lectures and demonstrations, through sensational events such as the post-mortem on Sara Baartman (the Hottentot Venus), high-profile operations to separate conjoined twins, and the highly theatrical mummy unwrappings. Even so, the great mystery of heredity and its mechanisms remained unsolved until 1900 (when Mendel's work was rediscovered); and this, paradoxically, may have contributed to theatre's fascination with it, as the question of how traits were passed on was still wide open and therefore subject to all kinds of speculation, debate and representation.

Ibsen gets away with some rather shaky medical explanations for the hereditary diseases afflicting his characters (e.g. Dr Rank in *A Doll's House*, Oswald in *Ghosts*). His plays rehearse common misconceptions, like the idea that alcoholism can be inherited or that one can develop syphilis from overindulgence in truffles and champagne – though of course such medical vagueness is also a neat way of evading stage censorship. As his plays also increasingly shift the emphasis on diagnosis of a disease rather than its cure, they become crucial elements in the training of the audience's diagnostic gaze. Specifically, we are trained to examine psychology, a new branch of medicine and science with its own methods, which audiences needed to learn. Watching an Ibsen play meant trying to understand first the problem or condition affecting the characters, then the underlying causes of it; not, however, solving or curing it, usually because such a thing doesn't exist (yet). Freud remarked of Ibsen that what makes him a 'great dramatist' is that he 'loves to pursue problems of psychological responsibility with unrelenting *rigour*' (Freud, 1916, 379; my emphasis). It is not just that he pursues such problems, it is that he does so with rigour – a prized attribute and requisite feature of any medical professional.

Yet, just as the rise of psychology as a discrete field of study in the late nineteenth century was signalling a delving inward, eugenics – which emerged at exactly the same time – was giving new emphasis to the visible, to the ways in which inner, mental 'unfitness' could be manifest in the face and the body (Wolff, 2009).

Eugenics suggested that invisible goings-on inside the mind and visible physical conditions alike were texts that could be read, interpreted and performed. It cloaked its spurious methods and biases in the respectability of medical diagnosis. This is a key development in the diagnostic gaze of the audience, and it comes during a period of 'revolutionary advances in medical technologies for penetrating, measuring, and representing the body; for reconstructing and extending it prosthetically; and for treating its states of disease' (Garner, 2008, 313). The new invasiveness came about through X-ray, anaesthesia and improved surgical techniques, and they provided potent metaphors for theatrical naturalism. In his 1878 manifesto for naturalism in the theatre, Emile Zola exhorts dramatists to dissect and anatomize; by 1897 Bernard Shaw can write of the 'pathologic horrors' with which realism had, by this time, become associated – as if that was all it offered (Shaw, 1897, 12).

Naturalism, says Zola, is 'the expression of our century' (in Zola 1878 reprinted in Worthen, 1995, 1182–6). His famous essay has tended to be read in terms of science, particularly biology and anatomy, as he exhorts theatre to become more scientific, just as Brecht would do in his essays for a 'scientific theatre'. It is true that he hails 'experiment' in theatre just as in the sciences, and that he talks of the nineteenth century as a period of 'inquiry and analysis'. As he puts it, 'we are an age of method, of experimental science; our primary need is for precise analysis' (Zola in Worthen, 1995, 1183). But his concern with 'physiological man' also suggests a specifically medical context for such analysis. He casts the history of the theatre not just as a dramatic 'evolution' but as an afflicted body. Naturalism comes from 'the very entrails of humanity' (1181). Thus, in this bodily metaphor, theatre is growing more organic, moving from the superficial and external (he sneers at the doublets and togas of classical tragedy) to the internal and physiological with its new focus on heredity, the workings of the mind and the mysteries of the body. The 'enfeebled', 'exhausted' and impotent theatre will be 'revived' through naturalism, a form of playwriting that takes 'the thoroughgoing analysis of an organism' as its objective, and shows characters whose 'muscles and brain[s] function as in nature' (1184). Such plays are 'pulsing with life' (1184) because they 'burrow … deeply into humanity' (1185).

Seeing Zola's essay in light of medical discourse opens up new meanings not offered by reading it solely in terms of science. It shows Zola moving freely between the perspective of both doctor and patient, conceptualizing theatre as performing both roles. The hinge for both perspectives is diagnosis founded on close observation. A thorough-going criticism of contemporary cultural forms is being launched in the latter half of the nineteenth century, calling for a new art, theatre and literature based on the methods of medicine.

Medical men

To illustrate comprehensively the rich and layered engagement between nineteenth-century medicine and theatre is not possible here, but I would like to provide some snapshots in the form of representative plays chosen not because they deal with doctors on stage – that is a different topic – but because they give insights specific to their times about the public conception of medicine.[3] In different ways, they 'express the nature of our contemporary intelligence' as Zola put it in his essay (Zola, 1995, 1182), although 'intelligence' hardly seems an apt term to apply to W.S. Gilbert's one-act 'comedietta' A Medical Man: this slight, utterly forgettable piece suggests a certain conception of the medical profession, but it is also of interest for making comedy out of the central conceit of merging the seemingly distinctive domains of theatre and medicine.

Alphonso de Pickleton, an unsuccessful young playwright who is waiting for a visit from the theatre manager considering his sensational drama 'Patriarch and the Precipice, or the Blue Pill of Despair', pretends to be a doctor in order to impress Belinda, a lovely young lady who has just pretended to fall down the stairs and land unconscious outside Alphonso's flat in order to lure him to her aid and eventually catch him for a husband. She knows he is only pretending to be a doctor but she plays along. All of the usual clichés are here: the writer as shy, hapless and untidy; the 'medical man' as authoritative, impressive and virile. In his guise as a doctor, Alphonso becomes quite eloquent; he tells her that she has sustained

> an exceedingly ugly fall, and it's impossible to say what the consequences may be...Exposure for one moment to the open air might, and probably would, induce rheumatic ossification of the pericardiac sal ammonia! Think how dreadful that would be! (Gilbert, 1870, 25)

Donning the authority of a doctor does Alphonso good, as he tells the audience in an aside: 'Well, for a bashful man, you're getting on.' And all it takes is a bit of pseudo-medical jargon. He then offers amputation: 'If you'd like a leg whipped off, I'll do it in a jiffey. Do have a leg off!' (Gilbert, 1870, 26) In fact, he tells her, she is in the very room where he carries out such procedures; 'not half an hour ago I whipped off three legs and an arm in the very chair you're sitting in' (26).

Medical professionalism soon melts into a profession of love. But they are interrupted by Jones, the theatre manager, who has come to complain about Alphonso's play. Alphonso pretends that Jones is one of his patients, and a slew of medical puns ensues:

> Jones I've called about this 'Blue Pill' of yours. Do you know, I'm afraid I can't take it.
> Alph Can't take it? Nonsense! Why not?
> Jones Why, in the first place, there's a great deal too much of it.
> Alph Too much of it? Why, what do you mean?
> Jones Why, I mean that I don't think it will go down. I'm quite sure it wouldn't be long in the bill.
> Alph Never you mind whether it will be long enough in the bill; the question is, whether you're broad enough in the throat.
> Jones Broad enough in the throat? I don't understand you, sir.
> Alph Yes, for it to *go down*. It's a joke. (Gilbert, 1870, 27–28)

The banter (which continues for many more minutes) follows the standard pattern of vaudeville cross-talk, with its repetition of punch lines and setting up of puns. It conflates two separate domains by overlaying theatrical jargon with medical terms, delighting in their unexpected commonality (how will the pill/the play 'go down'). Alphonso advises Jones to 'take it at once' and Belinda chirps up that it would do Jones 'a great deal of good' and that Alphonso 'must know better than you'. But Jones is adamant; the leading actress is 'determined to throw it up' (Gilbert, 1870, 28–29). This goes on until the inevitable moment of revelation of Alphonso's true identity to Belinda. She feigns outrage at being thus deceived, and in his defence – the speech that closes the play – he asks rhetorically, since he has brought about such happiness and healing (giving Jones a successful play, making Belinda happy through his love, making himself happy by acquiring Belinda): 'Am I not…justified in describing myself as a singularly successful Medical Man?' (Gilbert, 1870, 36).

This light comedietta articulates several key questions about the status of medicine at this time: the easy slippage between medical authenticity and charlatanism, the Jonsonian gullibility of the public, theatre and medicine's shared basis in performance, and the common ground between divergent disciplines. These strands all emerge again very strongly, and in much sharper satire, at the turn of the century in Shaw's *The Doctor's Dilemma* (1906). In the opening scene, Shaw pokes fun at the medical profession's ability to capitalize on its own failures. Two doctors reminisce about 'the woman with the tuberculosis ulcer on her arm' whom one of them attempted to cure with Koch's tuberculin, 'and instead of curing her, it rotted her arm right off…Poor Jane! However, she makes a good living out of that arm now by shewing it at medical lectures' (Shaw, 1906, I, 507). This signals the play's thorough-going attack on the medical profession as ruthlessly, amorally exploitative. The same gulling of the patient through medical jargon that Gilbert had fun with in his *Medical Man* is evident throughout Shaw's play, as in Walpole's development of a lucrative business in removing the 'nuciform sac' from well-to-do patients – an entirely fictional organ that he alleges causes lethal blood poisoning. Like most of the other doctors in the play, he is a well-educated charlatan, extracting money by playing with people's lives for his own gain; that he is part of an elite medical profession, rather than a fairground charlatan, makes him especially culpable.

This is the main target of the play's polemic, but Shaw also tackles other issues. The play questions how medical progress is channelled and manipulated by doctors. It suggests that not everything deemed a breakthrough is a step forward, and indeed it may even have been thought of before and roundly dismissed. It posits that old-fashioned methods are better than new ones, going so far as to wax nostalgic about the blessed days *before* chloroform: 'in my early days, you made your man drunk; and the porters and students held him down; and you had to set your teeth and finish the job fast' (Shaw, 1906, I, 508–9). Doctors and patients used to be made of sterner stuff; modern medicine is effete, pandering and etiolated. The play even posits mischievously that pioneering medical discoveries cause more damage than good. But Shaw was swimming against the tide and he knew it, watching as medical authority was gaining greater power. The staying power of the play is its central suggestion that all of medicine is self-consciously performative. The doctors perform for each other, vying for patients and prestige. Medical breakthroughs are performances that get applauded and rewarded. The plodding country doctor is dull because he is unobserved, just going about his routine work. In this context, it is worth noting that even Darwin's father, a dedicated and scrupulous doctor, defined success as a doctor in terms that bring to mind Shaw's satire: 'exciting confidence' and '[getting] many patients' (De Beer, 1983, 25). Shaw's play exposes how far that word 'confidence' has changed to its other meaning of tricking ('confidence-men') as the old system of trust and 'confidence' has eroded into one of manipulation and extortion; and how far the medical profession, newly professionalized, needs regulation. Indeed, the play's implicit plea for nationalized health care is one of the many reasons for its continued relevance.

The Doctor's Dilemma is based on several actual events and people, chief among these the colourful and controversial Sir Almoth Wright (later nicknamed Sir Almost Right with regard to penicillin). Wright sent Shaw a pamphlet in 1905 on tuberculosis inoculation and invited him to visit his laboratory. On one visit, Shaw sat in on a late-night lab break when a discussion arose over whether to admit a new patient just arrived that day for treatment using a new experimental method, and Shaw asked: What would happen if more people applied to you for help than you could properly look after? Wright said: We should have to consider which life was worth saving. Theirs was a mutually beneficial relationship:

Wright saw Shaw as a great advertisement for his vaccine therapy; Shaw saw Wright as a way of combating the superstition that a playwright cannot be a biologist (Holroyd, 1989, 164).

Henry Arthur Jones' *The Physician* (1897), which like *The Doctor's Dilemma,* opens in posh consulting rooms and features a successful doctor (Carey) confiding in the older country doctor: 'I want to consult you about myself' (Jones, 1897, n.p.). He doesn't know what's wrong; says he has 'a horrible despair in his heart'. Shaw echoes this almost exactly in *The Doctor's Dilemma* when Ridgeon confides in Sir Patrick in the opening moments of the play that he has 'a curious aching' and doesn't know what is causing it (Shaw, 1906, I, 508). In *The Physician*, this curious aching is self-diagnosed: Carey thinks he has 'caught the disease of our time, our society, our civilization.... Middle age. Disillusionment. My youth's gone. My beliefs are gone. I enjoy nothing. I believe in nothing' (Jones, 1897, n.p.). He wants 'a new impulse, a new outlook on life – no, I want a new life itself', but says that he still has the 'healing instinct strong within' him so that 'if any poor devil suffering from some mortal disease were to come in at that door and ask me to help him, I should fling myself heart and soul into his case and fight like a tiger to pull him through' (Jones, 1897, n.p.). Moments later, such a desperate soul does come in: an alcoholic who is beyond cure but whose pleas for help Dr Carey cannot ignore; so he's found his new cause, and the rest of the play shows him devoting himself to trying to cure the patient while falling hopelessly in love with the patient's betrothed, just as Ridgeon does with Dubedat's wife in *The Doctor's Dilemma*. The patient conveniently dies in the end, leaving the way clear for Carey to marry the woman, who of course has narrowly escaped being infected with the disease of alcoholism herself as she was just on the verge of marrying the doomed man. There are several striking parallels here with Shaw, but *The Doctor's Dilemma* makes more sharply unconventional fare out of Jones's materials by clothing allusions to real-life medical research and practice in polemical discourse and theatricality.

Another key influence on Shaw was French playwright Eugene Brieux, whom he championed at a time when plays like *Damaged Goods* (1901), which dealt frankly with syphilis, were being refused a license by the Lord Chamberlain. Another of his plays that has received little attention actually connects more directly with

Shaw's concern with doctors. Brieux's *Les Remplaçantes* (1901) is, improbably, a play entirely about wet-nursing (though without once showing the act of breastfeeding, which all takes place offstage or discreetly behind screens). It was surprisingly successful at the time and it contains a sub-theme of city versus country doctor, very much a theme in *The Doctor's Dilemma*. Its main target, however, is the medical and political collusion in the scandalous French wet-nursing system, by which poor country girls left their own babies (usually born out of wedlock, though significantly not in Brieux's play) and went to work as wet-nurses in Paris amongst wealthy mothers who were afraid their elegant figures would be ruined by breast-feeding. The money the country girls earned rarely made it intact back home to support their babies, as it passed through the hands of the pimp-like mayors who farmed the girls out, or was frittered away by self-indulgent husbands, partners and families back home. There is much earnest discussion between the two main doctors in the play about this problem, and the play comments extensively on the dynamic between urban and rural medicine. But the play, like many of Brieux's others, is so thorough in its diagnosis of societal ills that it forecloses and frustrates the audience's own diagnostic gaze. Perhaps this, more than criticisms of poor dramaturgy or dull dialogue, is what has relegated Brieux's drama to the museum of theatre history and the arena of academic study.

Finally, and staying with France for the moment, I want to look at how some of the things Shaw targets in the medical profession were to be dramatized by an unusual playwright: doctor Henri de Rothschild, who wrote almost forty plays in the latter half of his life under the pseudonym of André Pascal. The great-grandson of the founder of the Rothschild wine and banking dynasty, he was an extraordinarily active and energetic doctor, scientist and playwright whose medical work had a lasting impact in ways that we now take completely for granted. He pioneered the field of paediatrics and the science of infant feeding, he set up maternity hospitals in Paris and the provinces, and spent huge sums of his own money financing experiments to find better ways of treating severe burns (Paul, 2011). Likewise, he financed the building of a small theatre and the production of his plays there. These two careers – the medical and the theatrical – overlapped: Rothschild continued to work as a doctor and scientist while writing plays that dealt with medical and scientific themes. Almost all of his plays (some written with collaborators) are now forgotten, but they received attention at the time and they are notable for trying to dramatize issues about the medical profession that are still relevant today. For example, Rothschild observed, and was troubled by, pervasive and exploitative problems in French medicine, namely 'le charlatanisme' of so much of French medical practice and the widespread system of fee-splitting ('la dichotomie'), whereby doctors often needlessly referred patients to their surgeon friends and shared the resultant fees. These issues went into plays such as *Le Caducée* (written in 1910, published in 1912, and revised and performed in 1921), often seen as his best theatrical work, and *Le Grand Patron* (1931), which made a 'big splash in the world of Parisian theater' when it opened at the Comédie des Champs-Elysées (Paul, 2011, 231).

In addition to the ethical issues they raise, such works of the early twentieth century highlight another aspect to the changing relationship between medicine and performance: the crystallizing of all of medicine into the metonymic figure of the white-clad (and predominantly white male) doctor. In fact, medical men were only a part of a much larger canvas. Nineteenth-century medicine was signified in performance by a greater range of roles, including most prominently the midwife and the nurse – Florence Nightingale, 'the lady with the lamp', being only the most visible example, an iconic image that pervaded Victorian culture. By the time of Shaw, Rothschild, Sean O'Casey in *The Silver Tassie* (1927), or Sidney Kingsley in *Men in White* (1933), for example, the nurse has taken second place to the white-coated doctor and the midwife is virtually unseen. Part of O'Casey's play is set in a hospital; Harry, former football star and local hero, now uses a wheelchair and is embittered after being wounded in combat in the First World War, reduced as he puts it to a 'shrivelled thing' (O'Casey, III, 231). The callous doctor, Surgeon Maxwell, eventually insists that he be taken home due to his extreme emotion: 'we can't have this sort of thing going on', 'bring the boy home, woman, bring the boy home' (O'Casey, IV, 246). *The Silver Tassie* is fundamentally an anti-war drama, but it also asks questions about the limits of medicine, and it suggests that a dry-eyed, realistic and ultimately pragmatic approach works best. It is especially striking how the character of Susie gains 'dignity and a sense of importance' from becoming a nurse (O'Casey, III, 219). It is she who utters the final thoughts on Harry's future: disabled veterans like him 'have gone to live their own way in another world. Neither I nor you can lift them out of it…. We can't give sight to the blind or make the lame walk', and the able-bodied must simply carry on living without them (O'Casey, IV, 248). The play's chilling depiction of medical treatment and a medical establishment that is wholly ineffective and uncaring retains strong traces of *The Doctor's Dilemma*.

In treating all of these different examples in one discussion, I am aware of the risk of flattening important cultural distinctions; after all, the medical systems of Britain, France and Norway are hardly one and the same. One also has to be cautious about ascribing lofty motives where there may be none; while it is true that Shaw takes the medical profession thoroughly to task in *The Doctor's Dilemma*, his impulse to write the play came simply from a challenge by his friend the theatre critic William Archer saying in an article that Shaw was unable to write a convincing death scene (Holroyd, 1989, 167). Gilbert provided *The Medical Man* for critic Clement Scott's collection of 'drawing-room plays' aimed at proving that theatre could get beyond the usual fare of simpering heroines and sentimental plots. Yet they – like so many other plays and performances of their times and across cultures – collectively demonstrate how theatre's engagement with medicine often reveals, in varying degrees, an uneasiness about the unbridled power of doctors, who was regulating them, and how the public could penetrate their specialized discourse, diagnose their failings, or see into their private world of privilege. These issues have, if anything, sharpened in the public consciousness and theatre remains an important site for their exploration and articulation, as recent plays like Peter Nichols' *The National Health* (1969), Lucy Prebble's *The Effect* (2012) and Nina Raine's *Tiger Country* (2011) demonstrate. Whether consciously or not, such plays build on and continue the multi-faceted and complex legacy of nineteenth-century medical and performance interconnections.

3

The Bluer Flowers of the Medical Theatre: Visiting with Aliens, Poppies and Antipodean Spas

Petra Kuppers

How do you travel? How do you visit far away, and close by? This is what Walter Benjamin asks of us:

> [W]alk out your front door as if you've just arrived from a foreign country; to discover the world in which you already live; to begin the day as if you've just gotten off the boat from Singapore and have never seen your own doormat or the people on the landing... – it is this that reveals the humanity before you, unknown until now. (Benjamin, 1999, 427)

This chapter uses Benjamin's invitation in the *Arcades Project* as a lens to think about an international *flânerie*. Join me as I go travelling, as a disabled performance scholar and artist. Benjamin offers me scenery, costume-chests and make-up to see some of the stranger theatres of medical performance at work, in semi-publics, in hidden places, on the edge of the street.

In previous publications, I have analysed how artists dealt creatively with diagnoses and their narratives, subverted the diagnostic gaze, and made performances at the edges of art and science. In this chapter, my performance lens focuses on art/life with a smaller 'a', not material created for galleries or theatres, but a more everyday kind of joyful engagement with cultural scenes. This engagement is similar to Benjamin's embodied analysis of what it means to be an urban person in modernity. Benjamin 'botanizes on the asphalt', walks as a *flâneur* through the city, privileged and invisible, and his artful meandering has influenced cultural studies types ever since.

Over the years, we have critiqued the privilege of the *flâneur*, have called ourselves *flâneuses*, and have articulated race, class, gender, sexuality and disability into the city scenarios. But this method of knowing remains juicy and seductive: going for a walk while keeping one's senses open and reading one's embodied performance against the registers of cultural critique. The world becomes a theatre, and the surreal art/life gaze falls where it will.

In the main part of Benjamin's *Arcades Project*, small scenes and cultural texts on life in Paris create a rich tapestry. One of these scenes speaks to the ways that Parisian urban life brings together interior private settings, facades and public displays. In this little narrative here, Monsieur Chabrillat is the director of a Parisian theatre, who inherits a wax museum. Chabrillat:

> is friends with a certain bohemian, a gifted draftsman, who at the time is homeless. This man has an idea. Among the waxworks in this museum is one group representing the visit of Empress Eugenie to cholera patients in Amiens. At the right, the empress smiles on the patients; to the left is a Sister of Charity in white cornet; and lying on an iron cot, pale and emaciated beneath the fine clean bedclothes, is a dying man. The museum closes at midnight. The draftsman opines: Nothing simpler than to remove, with due care, the cholera patient, lay him on the floor, and take his place in the bed. (in Benjamin, 1999, 408)

The artist in the museum, taking the place of the sick mannequin to cover up homelessness, with empress and sick-nurse watching over cholera – there seems rich juice for me, here, to revisit some of the core ideas of the *Arcades Project*, all themes which I will weave into my own embodied medical *flânerie*.

Benjamin identifies three mechanisms of the arcade aesthetic. First, modernity transplants privacy into the public and back again. Second, illusionary class mobility becomes a mechanism of healing. Third, 'antiquity' is always just before or after the current moment, asserting the 'contemporary' moment's monumentality. These three themes all, in different ways, relate to issues of medical embodiment and performance, too. So here, I will excavate these moments and link them to my own travel *flânerie*, illuminating aspects of medical art/life.

Private publics

In the Claretie passage, the public display in the wax museum becomes a place of the uncanny home, a place to sleep, to give one's self to the nightly roaming of dreams. This mechanism, the interpenetration of public and domestic, is central to Benjamin's *Arcades Project*: Wilhelmian house facades create niches that invite passers-by into domesticity, the steel and glass of the arcade echoes both futuristic commerce, and utopian communal living arrangement in which no energy is wasted. The wax museum partakes in this in-between status: it is both beholden to the older pre-categorizing knowledge machine of the Wunderkammer and chimes with democratizing ambitions that make the elevated life human and everyday.

As a site of medical performance, the wax museum fulfils multiple functions, from horror to pleasure and back again. It holds the horrors and titillation of the waxen simulacra of warts and wounds, scabs and prostheses well known from the more arcane displays of the Mütter Museum in Philadelphia and the Hunterian Museum in London. But horror is close to other affects: the wax museum is also the place of seduction, of vicarious pleasure, of scopophilia and erotic awakening.

Siegfried Kracauer, another German modernist writer, calls upon his own teenage memory of the wax museum in the arcade, of medical performance in the most direct sense: the site of the woman's body, an anatomical specimen, cut for medical display (1992, 49–55). The place of window-shopping becomes the place where body as experience and image meet. Here, in the anatomy museum, a boy could get acquainted with the mysteries of the human body, and in particular, the female body. Kracauer writes that at this arcade, a doctor demonstrated an anatomy session to curious onlookers, excavating the organs out of a waxen female body.

Disgust and (horrifically displaced) attraction: the street and the wax museum are emblematic sites of vision as consumption, making women's bodies into objects of revulsion and titillation at the same time.

Upward mobility

The two female figures stand above the sleeping artist – a nun, pointing heavenward, and an empress, pointing to another elevated station that never quite went out of fashion, even in post-revolutionary Parisian times. These two women seem to be symbols of passages more than entities in their own right, they point to the act of travelling, to going up high. This is a feature Benjamin points to many times in the *Arcades Project*: contact with the old aristocracy becomes its own healing for the nostalgic petit-bourgeois. In a later passage, this magical healing bestowed by the empress appears again, in reference to mineral springs. Koch writes of the poems dedicated by Goethe to Maria Ludovica at Karlsbad:

> The essential thing for him in these 'Karlsbad poems' is not the geology but…the thought and the sensation that healing energies emanate from the otherwise unapproachable person of the princess…in the presence of the mystery of the springs, health comes…from the proximity of the princess. (in Benjamin, 1999, 413–4)

To partake in spa culture is to touch elevated life, a vanished life of either antiquity or aristocracy. This memory of elevation becomes one of the healing dreams of modern man (with women usually in the position of the exalted others, not enjoying their own bath).

This is a medical performance of well-being, of spa therapy, the magic of being removed from the everyday toil in the warm waters and gracious curves of marble tubs. Intimacy and emanations: well-being emerges from an intimacy that is hard to come by in the cities where beds might be shared with dead wax figures.

Monuments

That poor sleeper escaped quite nicely from poverty: it's whom you know, not what you know. The relationality of the city assured him a sleeping place, even if he first has to move a waxen dying man aside. The artist's name is not recorded here, though: the men (and women) of the *Arcades Project* are usually nameless, unless they happen to be Baudelaire, Goethe, or theatre directors, and anonymity is one of the plagues of modern life in the mass. So in a third mechanism, Benjamin points to another device the bourgeois uses to assert his right to being remembered: touching the ancients. For the touch of the ancients, qua being ancients, assures that memory itself is possible. Importance, here, is homeopathically bestowed, and the touch of old marble busts might ensure that one's own likeness might eventually find a place in a museum or a history book.

The artist, of course, sleeps among wax figures, creatures ready to melt away at a torch's touch. Throughout the *Arcades Project*, the commodified, fetishized, voyeuristically attained, *flânerie*-found object recedes, and melts into thin air.

I have identified three movements in Benjamin's work, all focused on the displaced and displacing artist of the mobile economy, who sleeps beneath the women angels. I will now travel a bit further, as another artist/scholar on the road, looking for a place to put her head, and store her wheelchair for the night.

Private publics: Reading weeds

The first of the three contemporary medical performance sites of this chapter is in Aotearoa/New Zealand. It is a visual art intervention in a damaged city, a healing for urban space and people, through the power of an ancient medical system: medicinal plants and botany. I am in Christchurch, a city deeply disrupted by the deadly earthquakes of 2010 and 2011.

The Re:START mall is all around me, a container city of shops and food trucks. It is chichi, and pretty, brimming with life on a Wednesday afternoon, tourists and locals mingling at all the outdoor tables. The container aesthetic meets life hacking meets neoliberal marketplace of hip newness. Walking around in this field, I encounter strange flowers, literally. On a black wall next to a container that houses a temporary office of the ANZ, an Australian/New Zealand bank, two half-peeling posters arrest me with their delicacy, and their non-shiny, non-new appearance.

Variations*Order is a Botanical Preservation Project, part of The Social, a social practice artists' collective working in Christchurch for a few years now, charting redevelopment and emergence in their own way:

> The core of our practice has everything to do with critical public dialogue and setting up environments for social connections to take place within the urban centre of a post-quake city. (from The Social tumblr)[1]

Artist Liv Worsnop, in an interview at the Hummingbird Café, tells me about how she created the delicate images on those peeling posters that arrest my city *flânerie*. One of the images is a scan of a pressed California poppy, a settler in New Zealand soil, and, I am sure, a well familiar figure in Benjamin's Paris.

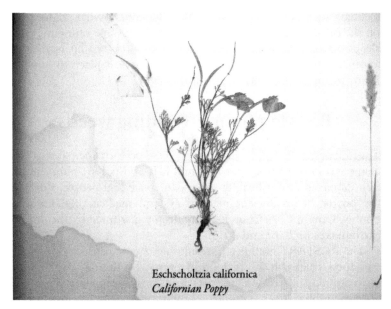

Eschscholtzia californica
Californian Poppy

FIGURE 3.1 *Poppies. Photo by Petra Kuppers.*

The image is pale green and delicate pink, not at all the brash colours that I personally associate with the popping poppy of California. This flower is much more ethereal, cleaned of all soil, free floating, a traveller on a creamy white field. The seed pots arch outwards like spears, elegant and balletic. The flowers look papery, like tissue, semi-translucent. Where two petals overlap, their colour briefly intensifies, as if in solidarity with one another.

This text appears on the poster:

Eschscholtzia californica
  Californian Poppy
  NZ Naturalization – 1878
  From America
  MEDICINAL: Californian Poppy has been shown to be a soporific herbal remedy. Experiments have shown it to act like morphine. It has been used as a sedative and to induce sleep.
  HOMEOPATHICALLY: It is used to treat accelerated respiration, complete paralysis of the limbs, nervousness and restlessness and insomnia due to anxiety and worry. Californian Poppy supports and stabilizes a balanced process of spiritual and moral development by encouraging more self-responsibility and quiet inner development.

Layers and layers of meaning overlap, like the petals: caring for a city, caring for biological entities, travel across seas from different continents, altered states and reminders of the panic of the quakes, the direct physical effects of what it might have been like to find one's self physically threatened, to know loved ones are dying or injured, to be thrown to the ground.

What ails, what cures, what price is to be paid for the self-care that re-establishes equilibrium, a re-arrangement with what is 'real' and 'solid' is this floating Laputa? More 'self-responsibility': in the vision of clean redevelopment, who is excluded, who is homeless, and where are the new sites where those deemed unsightly, like the soil that might stick to roots, might re-settle?

Many of the social practice artists around Christchurch work with sarcastic tones, both invite and analyse 'being social', and what that may mean for different parts of this post-colonial, classed and stratified society in upheaval. Some of these social practice engagements feel quite easy to swallow: sanitized graffiti practices, a skateboarding place with clearly defined boundaries.

This eco-art project seduces me with its open boundaries, the field of cream and the floating signifiers of its plants. These seeds can grow in many directions, a medical performance of homeopathic influence or rhizomatic growth.

In the Variations*Order project, I can only find one native plant, Jersey Cudweed or Pukatea. All others are 'naturalized'. They come from elsewhere. The native plant was found in a rubble field at the corner of Colombo Street and St Asaph Street. The plant image shows two stacks, arranged in a semicircle leaning into each other, a shape vaguely reminiscent of the koru imagery, the curly abstracted shapes of ferns that grace much New Zealand branding, with its use of Māori patterns.

The flower heads are yellow and puffy, and they look fit to bursting with seed bodies ready to fly elsewhere. The description stresses dryness, brittleness and a fiery character:

> MEDICINAL USES: This plant is astringent meaning the herb draws together or constricts the body tissues and is effective in stopping the flow of blood. It is tightening, healing and drying on wounds. It can also reduce irritation and inflammation and create a barrier against infection …
> OTHER USES: Leaves are used as tinder.

There is a pucker in all the sweetness, flowers are astringent, too, not just sweet-smelling. Little nudges, mentions of irritation, find their way through the descriptions, through these decorative images displayed on the metal barriers that keep people out of the wild weed patches. Tinder: there is much that is smouldering under the bright façade of the Re:START mall.

The plant images also link themselves back to the Wunderkammer, an early forerunner of the museum, a chamber of wonders, akin and a kin to the wax museum of Benjamin's world. This library of thriving healing plants and peeling posters stands against the rational stacked order of the book-filled archive. Here, on the rubble strewn street corner, the library is destroyed, there is peeling paper, cream fields, and something more like the administering angels that watch over artists' sleep.

I feel myself touched by the quietness of the garden imagery, in Christchurch's self-reinventing Garden City, the non-shrill attention to life re-emerging. Cultural critique and an eye for beauty in all its forms need to keep a careful balance, and I am glad to rest for a while under the peeling poster, now already a year old, ready to fall down, like so much of Christchurch has done, to vanish into soil, and to bring forth new varied plants.

Upward mobility: Touching Venus

The next stop on my *flânerie* is in the desert, both near and far from urban space. It is tourist land, the outer edges of another city of angels, Los Angeles. I am in Joshua Tree Park, and I have driven my wheelchair-accessible van over rutted sand roads to an iconic site out here: the Integratron.

It rises before me in the desert, a round dome shiny and white against the ochre, orange and yellows of the surroundings. The

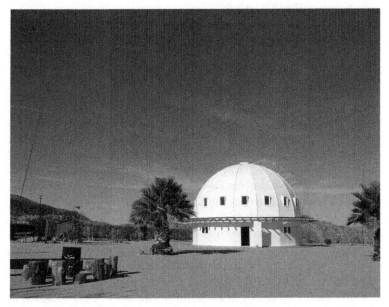

FIGURE 3.2 *The Integratron. Photo by Petra Kuppers.*

dome reminds me of observatories, cameras, rounded architectures that signify a reach towards knowledge. But there is no telescope inside: this round links us to the heavens in another way. The first descriptor on the Integratron's website already aligns many different systems of performing healing:

> This historical structure is a resonant tabernacle and energy machine sited on a powerful geomagnetic vortex in the magical Mojave Desert…Its creator, George Van Tassel (1920–1978), claimed that the structure is based on the design of Moses' Tabernacle, the writings of Nikola Tesla and telepathic directions from extraterrestrials. (from website)

Venusians, to be exact. Van Tassel received the blueprints for this dome and its functioning from visitors from Venus, and much of the building was financed by annual UFO devotee conferences. Now, the Integratron remains open to visitors for healing visits, and a daily performance of a sound bath explores the Integratron's most obvious feature: it's a perfect sound chamber. Three sisters are keeping the desert oasis alive, and they play an organ of crystal bowls to those of us lying in a circle on the wooden floor of the chamber, our bodies vibrated by the sounds and strange harmonics.

To be healed by the ultimate strangers, to be affirmed as important by those outside the scope of the familiar: what can be more emblematic of this modernist desire than Van Tassel's touch by alien hands? The site embraces a range of healing modalities much explored in nineteenth and twentieth century Paris and Berlin, too: the healing functions of energy and electricity, the magic of leylines and the science of telepathy. Contemporary medical performances draw upon these older modalities in multiple ways, and upon the relational magic of sleeping in tableaux: of co-dreaming in public, amplifying dreams with vibrations and sensory caress.

There is an order to how one approaches the sanctum. First, I am directed to the oasis that surrounds the dome. It is an artist garden, full of desert life, and with hammocks strung in star shapes around poles. Sofas sit in the desert sand that knows very little rain, and a water cooler ensures one's comfort. One has to book a space in everyday's performance, and even in mid-January, all is well booked up. Today, I am enjoying the calmness of the oasis, and sleep in a hammock for a while until I hear others arriving. We move past mirrors and welded art sculptures into the inner sanctum, a fenced ring around the white structure, and then, through a small door, into the cool interior. Do I feel it?

> The location of the Integratron is an essential part of its functioning. It was built on an intersection of powerful geomagnetic forces that, when focused by the unique geometry of the building, concentrate and amplify the earth's magnetic field. Magnetometers read a significant spike in the earth's magnetic field in the center of the Integratron. (from website)[2]

I do feel the coolness, and the ring of stillness that settles around this spatial concentration, this rounded shape in the middle of open space. I feel expanded and compressed as I make my way from the outer ring into the sanctum. Humans respond to spatial change, and my phenomenological sense of embodiment shifts when outer building skins layer me against the universe. There is a workout, of a kind, when moving through these gates and doorways.

Once inside, you have to walk up narrow and steep stairs. I leave my wheelchair behind and draw myself upward, providing a fun spectacle for others who might contemplate my spontaneous healing. I do walk in interior spaces, but to see an empty wheelchair is quite a sensation, as the signification of 'chair' is permanence and immobility. I imagine it is a bit like seeing a waxen cholera corpse suddenly flipping over the bed's edge. Up I scramble, part of the happily beaming crowd ready to step into the circle, take a brightly coloured woven mat and lie down to rest in a congenial circle of elevated ones.

I have not yet found particular references to aliens in the 1,000 pages of Benjamin's *Arcades Project*, this obsession being of a somewhat different age and space. But the glow of happiness and the elevation into heavenly spheres is certainly there, still at the bathhouse, the spa, the place of luxurious healing.

> Whereas a journey ordinarily gives the bourgeois the illusion of slipping the ties that bind him to his social class, the watering place fortifies his consciousness of belonging to the upper

class. It does this not only by bringing him into contact with feudal strata. Mornaud draws attention to a more elementary circumstance: 'In Paris there are no doubt larger crowds, but none so homogeneous as this one; for most of the sad human beings who make up those crowds will have eaten either badly or hardly at all ... But at Baden, nothing of the sort: everyone is happy, seeing that everyone's at Baden.' (in Benjamin, 1999, 414)

That is the draw of places like the Integratron, too. There is a mystery, and a happy one, one of plentitude and healing, and of being looked after in this giant cradle. Lying on the wooden floor, I can hear strange whispers: the people opposite me in the circle make sounds that amplify to me, and mine no doubt travel to them. I can hear alien breathing everywhere. It is disconcerting, but pleasant, a new hum, a flow of humanity louder than the already pretty loud hush that usually precedes a theatrical presentation when we notice the lights going down.

The introduction given is short, friendly, and does not mention much of the Venusian aspects of the building's heritage. The sounds that shortly begin to emanate from the struck and caressed crystal bowls do that labour all by themselves, no words needed. A sound bath. Crystals vibrating. Harmonics, resonating chambers in vibratory touch, exciting each other. Skin hairs, ear membranes, the bones of my face responding with minute movement. Sounds conducted via bone and air.

Richard Schechner has called performance 'restored behavior', twice-behaved behaviour, (2002, 29) and my critical reception here makes my body a tuning fork that links the spherical geometries (and sacred geometries) of so many of my healing journeys to my readings in the history of aesthetic engagements with space. I feel, and I think about feeling, and I feel that thinking affecting my ability to feel. I draw upon my meditation skills, and throw my anchors loose, to enter into once-behaved immediacy. I do really want to dissolve myself in the sound of the spheres, and I am reaching out, with my senses, to the magnetic field, to the leylines, to the stars.

Then someone starts snoring. Pretty soon, I feel the hardness of the floor beneath the colourful throw. I am back in the duration of the performance, and the moment vanishes.

Monuments: Embattled spa

My last medical performance moment is inside the spa, this iconic nineteenth/twentieth-century site of healing. I am in Aotearoa/New Zealand, in Rotorua, one of the Southern Hemisphere's centres for spa culture. I am here with Bree Hadley, a disabled theorist, and a fellow disabled woman who, like me, values the therapeutic effects of hot water: once behaved, and twice behaved, together. We are not just ironic quoters in the waters, we do experience the bliss of pain-free movement.

Before we immerse ourselves, though, we go to the museum: the right order of things for work and pleasure in modern individuals always ready to bow to the improvement yoke. The Rotorua Museum dedicates one of its wings to its history as a spa, and we can see original bath apparati and numerous photographs of long-dead Europeans who tried to merge Maori healing sites with European spa sensibilities. In these photographs, medicine becomes a performance: a posture, even an imposition, a caesura, a moment in time. Far from bringing universal medical truths to the colonies, the establishment found itself under attack from early on, having to defend 'therapy' in the light of a forward striding modernity that queries 'ancient wisdom', whether Maori or humoral theory.

New Zealand doctors had a very similar response to bath culture as Benjamin had, recognizing its European aristocratic/Roman antiquity aesthetics very nicely, and pushed back. The fact that Maori have used these healing springs for a long time seems to do little in assuaging the powers that be. Here is an excerpt from the Health Department's 1949 report that hastened the medical demise of the grand old spa at Rotorua:

> The old fashioned spa conception, a conception of treatment which has been responsible for the delayed knowledge of the treatment and cause of the rheumatic diseases – had to be abandoned, and the further exploitation of the mineral waters of Rotorua as miraculous cure-alls could not be condoned by the Health Department. A more rational and scientific outlook required to be developed (from Director of Physical Medicine, Dr G.A.Q. Lennane, written on boards inside old bathhouse. rooms, also on the Rotorua Museum website)[3]

So the spa and rest-cure culture of the sulphurous spring dropped off the official medical establishment's radar. But, like all the little Wunderkammers and their deliciousness, like the sound baths and their seduction, like all the other immersive pleasures of wax museums and vibration healing, it all survives. Travellers in matters of health create an alternative world, a slipstream to the official medical and scientific rationality, available to the botanizing world *flâneur*.

Spa-ing at Rotorua is alive and well, and of course it is a performance, too: the day we visited the 'official' big spa of Rotorua, we laid back and watched the crowds mingle. Tour buses full of Chinese tourists arrived, one after the other, and we observed, limbs heated from gorgeous silky waters and wrapped in towels, how people from cultures other than ours took to what to us was sacred quiet space. Conversation flew loud across the hot steam, and ladies in bathing caps started swimming laps in warm spring water. We laughed as the quietness of the Priest's Bath (so named after a priest who found himself miraculously cured of his joint pain when led to this old Maori spring) transformed into the bustling loudness of a Hong Kong evening.

We had travelled here, and travel had come to us, and different conceptions of how to perform health rituals were all around us. Balneology has not died, not in Europe, not in New Zealand, not in Asia. The spa no longer feels like being under the gentle touch of an empress, or under the thoughtful gaze of a nurse.

This spa does not have a very precious look, and I get little sense of touching the spheres. Instead, earth touches me: one of the other major exhibits in the Rotorua Museum is the history of volcanology in the region, the thermal earth currents that feed the healing waters, but that radically reshaped the region in the nineteenth century, destroying a Maori village and the thriving Pakeha/European tourist industry around it. This was one of the travel spots of the fashionable set, the bourgeois who might have wandered in the Paris arcades, too.

Lying in the spa pools, I can look out over the calm lake of Rotorua, and remember the many images in the museum and elsewhere, of people in waka (canoes) on the lake, the earth steaming and moving, the world transforming. Modernity undone, the dream of the arcades coming down. Steamed and wafting, between the volcano and the colonial adventure, the act of embodied reading feels alive.

Conclusion

[I]n the course of *flânerie*, far-off times and places interpenetrate the landscape and the present moment. When the authentically intoxicated phase of this condition announces itself, the blood is pounding in the veins of the happy *flâneur*, his heart ticks like a clock. (Benjamin, 1999, 419)

Modernity: hearts clicking like clock-work, I drive and fly hither and tither as a good modern privileged subject, freed from the bounds of her 'productive' labour by the vacation rights won by workers. In Benjamin's language, languor and bustle meet, they are two sides of the same coin, reliant on each other and interpenetrated.

I have travelled in this chapter, excavated multiplicities: private publics and their economies, freedom and (angel) patrons, cities and wilderness, health tourism and fads, the rhetorics of medico-health industrial complexes, neoliberal revitalization and gentrifying displacements. It *is* authentically intoxicating: there are moments when restored behaviour becomes immediacy, for a brief fleeting flash. And then I whip out the tourist camera and take my snap, and let my experience fall into what I know, into the passages of the *Arcades Project*.

My medical body performs its strata, its accretions, the layers of dirt in the city, and the accumulations of sulphur and salt on the spa tub walls. Reading the performances of my bodymind shows me the artfulness of living as a privileged patient, as a world-circling tourist. I lean into a modern antiquity – Benjamin's strata – to give me the pleasure of reading my experience. There are many steps of equivalency here, and I will stop parsing them now.

Benjamin's 1,000 page tome gives pleasure by allowing a writerly practice of reading to develop, giving space to an active reader to make her way through the citations and spatial moments. I think of this chapter as an invitation, too: reader, what are your medical adventures, your healing tourist anecdotes, and how can you shape your own artful weft? How does your authentic pleasure heighten itself through the artful repetitions and layerings of narrative? Living in conscious style, within the layers of precarity, chance and decay: this is an activating and active site of medical performance.

4

Performing Surgery

Roger Kneebone

The surgeon performed a delicate operation to repair a leaking heart valve.

Although the phrase 'performing surgery' is in common parlance, the emphasis is usually more on the surgery than on the performance. The earlier example would probably call to mind a sick patient with a diseased heart, not footlights and an applauding audience. Yet every operation *is* a performance, and such performances may be closer to the worlds of drama, dance, music and other performing arts than at first appears. In this chapter, I suggest that a shift of emphasis – from 'performing *surgery*' to '*performing* surgery' – can radically change what we see. Viewing surgery as an interplay of bodies – the body of the patient and the differently framed bodies of the surgical team – invites comparison with the craft of stage performance. Such a reframing poses new questions about boundaries and relationships (such as who are the performers and who the audience); about notions of expertise and skill; and about similarities and differences between domains, which at first seem incommensurable.

Much may be learned by comparison with other domains of expert practice. In order to unravel the idea of surgery as performance, I relate the closed 'insider' world of the operating theatre to performance outside the world of medicine, inviting wider interrogation. I explore how an enquiry which *sets out* to span apparently unconnected areas of practice may highlight areas that have become invisible to insiders, allowing them to see their world through an outsider's eye. While recognizing that the word 'performance' carries multiple meanings within specialized academic fields, I use the term in the lay sense most familiar to surgeons – that is, as the work of a performer (actor, dancer, musician) in a live encounter with an audience. As will be discussed, stage performer and surgeon both draw upon extensive training in order to carry out a series of learned actions, enacted within a collaborative setting, which are subject to unanticipated change.

In order to draw upon my own experience, I have written this chapter in the first person. A word of introduction may therefore be helpful. The first phase of my career was as a surgeon. After completing my undergraduate medical studies, I spent ten years training in general and trauma surgery, both in the UK and in Southern Africa. I then became a general practitioner, working for many years in a large group practice in Wiltshire, UK. In a third career change I became an academic and am currently Professor of Surgical Education at Imperial College London, with a special interest in simulation and engagement. These different, yet complementary, perspectives have convinced me of the value of cross-fertilization between domains of expert practice within and beyond medicine. In the process, however, they have provided more questions than answers. In this chapter I attempt to shape some of those questions.

I should point out that performing operations constitutes only part – though a crucially important part – of what surgeons do. Every aspect of clinical care – from consulting with patients and their families in preoperative clinics to providing postoperative care – depends upon expertise, and each involves some kind of performance. For this chapter, however, I focus on the operation itself.

The theatre of surgery

Of all the performing arts, theatre seems to offer the most immediate parallel. The terminology of surgery – 'performing' operations in an operating 'theatre' – has obvious resonances with the world of drama. Yet the question of 'what can surgeons and other performers learn from one another' sets an unorthodox frame of enquiry. For many surgeons, the idea that their work can be seen as performance at all – and that such performance might have parallels outside the world of medicine – can be uncomfortable. Those outside surgery, on the other hand, seldom have the opportunity to experience an operation from a clinician's perspective (as opposed to highly dramatized portrayals on film and television). After highlighting obvious points of correspondence between surgery and the theatre, I explore areas where the analogy starts to unravel.

To set the scene, I begin by describing key aspects of the surgeon's world. Even to outsiders, a surgical team is instantly recognizable. A group of gowned and masked figures surround a senseless form on the operating table. A huge circular lamp casts a brilliant beam. A hushed atmosphere is broken only by terse, softly spoken commands. Already there is tension and expectancy – the promise of cure set against the possibility of disaster. At centre stage the surgeon and his or her assistants are performing a procedure, using instruments passed by a scrub nurse. An incision surrounded by sterile drapes gives access to the patient's internal organs. At the patient's head stands the anaesthetist, surrounded by sophisticated technology, ensuring that the patient remains unconscious throughout the procedure and waking them up when it is over. Other figures move to and fro, adjusting equipment, fetching instruments and conveying messages.

The familiarity of this scene in popular culture masks its complex realities. Although, of course, there are dramatic, life-and-death moments, most surgery is routine and uneventful. As with stage performance, the skill which underpins surgery is not evident on casual inspection. Crucially, every operation depends on the seamless interweaving of expertise from many different backgrounds. Despite stereotypical portrayals of the heroic lone surgeon, surgery is never a solo performance. This fluid and seemingly effortless coordination of an expert team conceals years of rigorous training. Although patients may think and talk in terms of 'my surgeon', it is collaboration and team working that ensure the remarkable safety of most contemporary surgery.

Although framing surgery in terms of theatrical performance holds a seductive appeal, the comparison is more complex than it appears. If surgery is a performance, who is the audience and who the cast? And where is the patient in all of this?

It seems a truism to say that the primary focus of any operation must always be the patient. Yet in surgery, under general anaesthesia, the patient *as a person* disappears from view, as attention is narrowed to the physical aspects of the body. Although in one sense always central, in another the patient has been converted into a cipher or prop and bracketed out – only reappearing after the operation is over.

However, many complex procedures are now performed under regional or local anaesthesia. In such cases, the patient may indeed become an audience, acutely aware of the performance unfolding around them. Procedures involving the brain and its blood supply may not only allow but also *require* the patient to be conscious. In carotid endarterectomy (a procedure to remove fatty deposits from the main arteries to the brain), for example, the patient is prompted to talk throughout the operation so that the clinical team can monitor the brain's speech centres. This demands a reconfiguration of the patient's role, as audience member and active participant, as well as inert body (Kneebone, 2014). Surgery, therefore, takes place within a complex nexus of bodies, objects and representation (van Dijck, 2005), though this complexity may have become invisible to surgical teams themselves.

Surgery as performance

At each stage of an operation there are parallels with other kinds of performance, whether in terms of space, activity or people. As with performers in an opera or a play, participants come together in a specialized setting to which access is restricted. All must be dressed appropriately, changing out of their everyday clothes into 'costume' – patients into hospital gowns, surgical team members into 'scrubs'. From then on, surgery unfolds as a series of scenes. Once the operation has started, the spotlight moves (almost literally) from induction of anaesthesia to the procedure itself. The patient's skin is cleaned and draped, and the surgical team begin. Well-rehearsed steps are carried out in sequence, with surgeons and nurses working seamlessly as instruments move between them. At times, additional equipment, sutures or swabs may be required, whereupon an unscrubbed 'runner nurse' will fetch whatever is needed. A clear division of labour separates the functions of surgical, nursing and anaesthetic teams.

All of these steps are dominated by rituals and procedures. Although at one level these clearly have a scientific basis in bacteriology and infection control, they also have strong ceremonial – even hieratic – resonances. For example, 'scrubbing up' is a highly formalized process of hand washing and putting on a sterile gown and gloves, according to strict protocol. This allows those members of the team who will be touching the patient's body during surgery to remain sterile throughout the operation.

Scrubbing and gowning take place in an antechamber to the main theatre, where special sinks allow clinicians to go through a rigidly prescribed procedure. Yet, the scrub room is also a liminal zone, a space where team members can make the transition between states. Once in 'costume', surgeons assume an 'untouchable' status, protected both from physical contact and from distraction. The state of 'being scrubbed' entails walking in a particular way, hands clasped at chest height, skirting round potential contaminations and avoiding contact with unscrubbed colleagues. Like the dressing room, perhaps, the scrub room provides a quiet place where the ritual of putting on costume is integral to assuming a role, a character and a particular state of mind. Many surgeons describe this procedure as an opportunity to clear their mind of distractions, preparing themselves for the forthcoming operation.

Though this highly simplified account cannot begin to do justice to the complexity of surgery, it conveys a sense of a planned performance, carried out by highly trained experts. There is a division of labour; expert roles interdigitate; and explicit or implicit 'scripts' underpin a shared understanding of the team's purpose. Like the seemingly effortless improvisations of expert jazz musicians, success depends on teamwork and a collective memory of constituent practices.

Yet the theatricality of surgery, highly formalized and choreographed as it is, takes place largely outside the conscious awareness of its participants. Once the initial strangeness of the operating theatre has worn off, newcomers to surgery quickly assume the behaviours of those around them. Before long they start to conform to established 'ways of doing', no longer aware of what once appeared so strange. The 'reality' of carrying out actual surgery on a living person (rather than adopting a fictional role in a play) can obscure and conceal deeper parallels. Surgeons may not see their work as performance (in any theatrical sense) at all, but rather of 'doing work'. Indeed, for many clinical professionals, the word 'performing' carries undesirable overtones of entertainment and perhaps even frivolity.

So how might we make sense of surgery through such a lens? Shifting the focus from performing *an operation* (where the focus is the procedure itself and the frame is unquestionably medical) to performing as an activity in its own right, changes what is seen as criterial. Broadening the frame of performance to include surgery allows us to pose different questions about the nature of that performance. For example, we might ask what surgeons can learn from actors about assuming, then leaving, a role each time they go on stage. We might explore the process of negotiating the boundaries between one state and another – of being 'scrubbed', for instance. We might investigate how clinicians distinguish between performers and audience in a surgical setting, asking questions about the influence of being observed upon the practice of professionals from different disciplinary backgrounds. And we might ask what surgeons can learn about performance anxiety and dealing with adverse outcomes. This framing of performance as an abstracted study, removed from the instantiated forms of theatre, drama, surgery or whatever it may be, highlights new perspectives. Schechner, for example, writes of two meanings of performance: 'a showing of a doing and an activity demanding the coordinated efforts of a team working together at an extremely high level of skills' (Schechner, 2013, 214).

I argue that surgery is enacted by professionals according to strict rules, and that these resonate with other kinds of performance. For example:

- An operation, once started, must run until its conclusion.
- Participants in surgery have clearly defined roles and play parts within a broader enterprise.
- Those who carry out surgery do so in front of an audience (though it may be difficult to define exactly who this audience is).

- Every operation is unique, both in terms of the individual patient undergoing surgery and the team and conditions of its enactment.

- Successful surgery requires prolonged intensive training, effective teamwork, impeccable timing and the ability to respond appropriately to the unexpected.

- Flourishing as a member of a surgical team requires the ability to cope with the consequences of success and failure, using both praise and criticism to deepen insight and self-awareness.

- Although many operations are routine and surgery, generally, is extremely safe, the unexpected is always possible and disasters still occasionally happen. However extensive the preparation, nothing is entirely predictable.

Yet for all these similarities, there are marked differences. For example:

- Historically, surgeons have learned their craft by participating in actual operations – through performance rather than practice or rehearsal (though the prominence of simulation is challenging this view (Kneebone, 2009)).

- Surgery takes place in private, behind closed doors, while stage performance is designed for public consumption.

- The 'real' world of surgery is fundamentally different from the 'as-if' world of an opera or play. The consequences of error or failure are very different for patients and for audience members (Dieckmann et al., 2007).

- Feedback and criticism takes different forms.

Yet discussion between surgeons and performers is far from common, perhaps because people have simply not thought of making such connections. After all, becoming a surgeon, scrub nurse or anaesthetist – or a dancer, actor, comedian or stage magician – demands years of unremitting work. No wonder, then, that attention is focused on becoming an expert in a chosen domain, rather than reaching out to compare with others.

To many people, of course, surgical practice itself remains remote, though the *idea* of surgery exerts a powerful pull on the public imagination – at once alluring and repellent. Of course, surgery *as* performance has a history stretching back centuries, rooted in public dissections or 'anatomies'. With time, access to such spectacles became restricted. For decades, operating 'theatres' were built with viewing galleries (latterly behind glass). Yet these were for specialist audiences, for those with privileged access, for 'insiders' – medical students, visiting clinicians and so on. Recent technological developments are opening up surgery once more. The widespread presence of video cameras in operating theatres (prompted by keyhole surgery) is now expanding through YouTube, GoogleGlass and other approaches, allowing anyone to 'view' surgical procedures.

But for all this expanded accessibility, most views of surgery present operations that are already in the past and whose outcomes are known. Outsiders are invited to be spectators, not participants. Like watching the television replay of a Wimbledon final, something is lost if the performance is not live. Moreover, opportunities to *engage* directly with surgical teams and participate in their activities are few or non-existent. It is therefore very difficult to establish categories of correspondence between different worlds of performance as they are *experienced in the moment*. How then might it be possible to open up the closed world of surgery?

The secrecy of surgery

For obvious and excellent reasons, surgery takes place in private, behind closed doors. Controlling infection, maintaining confidentiality, ensuring security – all these require access restrictions. But at another level this hiddenness may have drawbacks. It means, for example, that those who are most affected by surgery – patients – may be least able to see what it involves, even if they want to. And it precludes other performers from exploring connections. Although surgery may need to be *hidden*, does this mean that its practices must remain *secret*? Might there be ways of *representing* that hidden world that capture the essence of its practices without trespassing on the originary world – the world of the actual operating theatre – itself? Might there be ways of inviting outsiders to experience performative aspects of surgery even though they have no medical training? And might it be possible to involve surgical teams in discussions (about performance preparation, say, or stage fright; about judging performance, or coping with negative critique and review) with experts from other domains?

In the following section, I outline my own work in creating *simulations* of surgery which bypass the protective 'force field' which surrounds clinical practice and repels outsiders.

Simulation

The concept of simulation is now firmly established within mainstream clinical education. Drawing on the familiar image of the aeroplane cockpit simulator, healthcare simulation sets out to recreate clinical practices without the possibility of causing damage. Using a combination of simple physical models, sophisticated computerized mannequins and a range of more or less realistic clinical settings, participants are able to practise aspects of their craft. At the simplest level, novices can repeatedly take blood from plastic arms. At the other end of the spectrum, entire clinical teams can rehearse their response to uncommon or potentially catastrophic events in a full scale, simulated operating theatre or intensive care unit. In many such simulations, trained actors (Simulated Patients) portray patients or clinicians (Nestel and Bearman, 2014). Simulation therefore occupies an interesting intersection between theatre and healthcare. In a practical sense, clinicians and educators are becoming more aware of the skills that professional actors can bring; at a metaphorical level, simulation provides a place of encounter between the different philosophical perspectives of clinicians and stage performers (Brodzinski, 2010).

A key benefit of simulation is that it offers protection from the consequences of error. No patient comes to harm and activities take place within an educational environment designed to support learning. Yet, although such facilities are widely available in many countries, high fidelity simulation is extremely costly in terms of space, resources and expert personnel. Simulation is therefore framed as a professional resource, designed and constructed for the training of doctors, nurses, paramedical professionals, educationalists and others and is almost as restricted as access to operating theatres themselves.

The following section outlines work by my multidisciplinary research group (the Imperial College Centre for Engagement and Simulation Science) in exploring alternative approaches to simulation aimed at overcoming these limitations. I propose that simulation can provide a point of entry through which those without medical training or traditional legitimacy can witness and participate in the practices of surgery. I argue that simulation – especially simulation of complex team settings, where skilled procedures are carried out under pressure – could provide a means for outsiders (whether they be patients, carers or other 'publics') to experience the processes of surgery. If successful, such engagement could lead to a deeper understanding for all concerned – a generous and respectful exchange in perspectives resulting in *reciprocal illumination*.

Innovation in simulation

For many years, my colleagues and I have been exploring how simulation might be used to recreate contexts of surgical performance (Kneebone, 2009). Distributed Simulation (DS), for example, refers to portable, low-cost simulation environments, which can be set up anywhere, without requiring the specialist facilities of a simulation centre (Kneebone et al., 2010; Kassab et al., 2011; Kassab et al., 2012). An inflatable enclosure can be erected in a few minutes, providing a 'surgical space' that represents the operating theatre or intensive care unit and selected 'props' represent key items of equipment. DS is based on 'selective abstraction', of identifying what is criterial in an originary world (here the world of operative surgery) and recreating a minimal, necessary set of contextual cues. These allow 'natives' of that world to work authentically with one another, while inviting non-specialist publics to observe and participate (Kneebone, 2010). This provides a 'working model' of a surgical setting, which can be manipulated without endangering actual patients.

The operations themselves are represented by realistic physical simulation, using theatrical prosthetics and/or haptic or virtual reality simulation technology. Performed by clinicians, procedures convey a vivid sense of what surgery entails, allowing experts and novices to experience the pressures and challenges of operating. Uncoupling realistic simulation from costly static centres has allowed us to experiment with different audiences and clinical conditions. Venues include science festivals, schools, museums, arts venues, public parks and music festivals. Conditions range from emergency abdominal and brain surgery to interventional cardiology for heart attack and treatment of adolescents with asthma.

In each instance, we have invited members of the public to participate as members of our clinical teams, working with clinicians to gain an insight into the processes of healthcare. This involvement of non-experts resonates with actual practice, where surgical teams are often augmented by inexperienced medical students who can still play a valuable part in assisting during operations. It is therefore possible to include members of the public and performers from domains outside healthcare in simulations, without compromising realism.

Case studies

It is against this background of realistic, portable, yet affordable simulation that we have worked with professional performers from other domains of expertise (including dance, classical music, jazz, magic and theatre). By inviting performers to *take part* in the activities of surgery, we have been able to explore their experiences in ways that would not have been possible otherwise. Simulation has provided a framework for sharing experience, and a common ground on which to base discussion of possible connections. The following brief descriptions summarize four recent case studies. Drawn from over ninety engagement and simulation events over the past seven years, these highlight the potential for cross-fertilization of ideas between apparently incommensurable areas of experience and expertise. Wider discussions with musicians, theatre performers, stage magicians, sportspeople and those from safety-critical industries, such as air traffic control and bomb disposal, have generated rich insights into aspects of practice which transcend disciplinary boundaries.

Improvisation in surgery

A collaboration with professional jazz pianist Liam Noble was prompted by observing a gig where his trio rapidly recovered from an unexpected mishap. It transpired that the manuscript sheet music (composed by Noble) in front of the bass player was out of synch with that of the other musicians. As soon as the bass player recognized the problem, he improvised a solution in the moment and the performance continued apparently unruffled. Subsequent discussions revealed marked similarities between the processes of jazz improvisation and the need for the surgical team to respond to unanticipated findings during the operation. Despite having no previous experience of surgery, Noble participated as a surgical assistant in a simulated operating team, and subsequent discussion explored areas of similarity.

Jazz improvisation and emergency surgery both depend upon 'pre-learned techniques linked together freestyle', allowing performers to tap into a reservoir of expertise shaped by experience (Twigger, 2010). The ability of clinicians and musicians to activate tacit and deeply embodied skills, almost without conscious awareness when responding to the needs of the moment, was especially striking (Kneebone, 2011). Subsequent conversations generated heightened awareness by surgeons and musicians of practices they had come to take for granted.

Surgery as a prompt for artistic response

A collaboration with choreographer Suba Subramaniam and dance group Sadhana Dance led to a fifty-minute performance inspired by the movements of clinicians in the operating theatre, *Under My Skin*.[1] Following initial discussion about the concept, Subramaniam observed live surgery at a large teaching hospital. Choreographer and dancers then took part in simulations of open and keyhole surgery led by experienced clinicians, drawing on this to create an artistic response inspired by surgery (rather than representing it directly). Extensive discussions during the preparation of the piece explored parallels and differences between dancers and surgical team members through an iterative development process. Discussions with audience members after each performance highlighted additional resonances. The dancers' focus on movement of bodies highlighted the interdependency of team members and drew attention to networks, which had become invisible to insiders.

Neurosurgery and a sculptor's eye

A simulation of neurosurgery for head injury showed a specialist surgical team drilling holes in the skull to relieve a blood clot. Sculptor Matthew Lane Sanderson, who participated as an audience member, then engaged with our team around parallels between his approach to materials and performance and the techniques employed by surgeons, raising technical questions that the clinicians had not previously considered. For example, Sanderson challenged the surgical team about their use of traditional techniques for performing craniotomy (removing a section of skull). This procedure involves drilling three circular holes in the skull, then connecting the holes with a miniature saw to create a triangular bone fragment that can be removed to give access to the underlying brain. Sanderson suggested that technology from engineering and woodworking might avoid the need for three holes and create only one, allowing surgeons to minimize bone trauma and speed up access. Framing neurosurgery as a procedure with strong similarities to creative artistry opened unexpected horizons of discussion, causing surgeons to rethink traditional ways of doing which they had previously accepted as a given.

The Scalpel and the Bow

A thirty-minute programme on BBC Radio 3 (2013) compared the experiences of string quartet players and surgical teams through sound (Kneebone and Williamon, 2013). Surgeons in training were audio-recorded while performing a challenging procedure (carotid endarterectomy) in high fidelity simulation. This procedure involves removing accumulations of fatty material (atheroma) from the carotid artery (which supplies the brain). In a parallel context, early career string quartet players were recorded while performing in front of a simulated audience. In each case, the 'inner voice' of selected participants (lead surgeon and cellist) was captured the following day in the audio. This inner voice was created through a process whereby each participant listened to a playback of their own recorded performance, then articulated their thoughts and feelings in the form of a spoken commentary overlaid upon the original recording.

In a later studio discussion, Kneebone and Williamon (Professor of Performance Science at the Royal College of Music) explored similarities and differences between these respective worlds. Issues such as performance anxiety and the need to block out distraction while retaining all-round awareness of other participants were evident in both groups of performers. This process of comparison highlighted the centrality of embodied knowledge, and the way in which the technical and procedural skills of an individual are expressed within a social context of performers working together to achieve a shared aim.

Though these brief descriptions raise more questions than they answer, they give a glimpse of how reciprocal illumination can lead to tangible changes in both artistic production and clinical practice.

Conclusion

This chapter has framed performance as an activity that transcends disciplinary boundaries. If framing surgery as a performance may invite new insights for all concerned, why has this not become more widespread? What is getting in the way? There seems to be a tension between practitioners and researchers. Practitioners (whether in surgery, sport or the performing arts) tend to stay within their frame of practice. Researchers, on the other hand, may explore comparisons within broad groupings, such as sports or the performing art; yet such framings seldom include surgery. Valuable opportunities for cross-fertilization are thereby overlooked.

It can be challenging for expert practitioners to look outside of their own arena of practice and explore commonalities with other experts, yet doing so can provide insight into the nature of expertise and prompt new ways of seeing what has become familiar. Simulation offers a means of bringing a closed professional world (in this case surgery) into view, inviting outsiders not only to observe but to participate. This shared physical experience has opened new possibilities for comparison and discussion. In the case of surgery, such connections may dramatically alter the way we see the body (whether that of the patient, clinician or both), making the familiar strange and opening new horizons of enquiry.

Despite the language of surgery – *performing* operations, working in an operating *theatre* – surgeons, in my experience at least, seldom *perceive* their work as performance. This reluctance has obscured opportunities for comparison. Yet the very uncertainties of such a framing – the challenges of establishing who are the performers, who is the audience and how such roles might unfold and be reconstituted – invite us to look differently at what we think we already know and ask ourselves new questions.

PART TWO

Performing Patients

5

The Patient Performer: Embodied Pathography in Contemporary Productions

Emma Brodzinski

Introduction

This chapter argues for the value of contemporary performance, as a practice that foregrounds the body, in countering received ideas of objectivity/subjectivity and passivity in the patient experience. It will focus on pathography in performance and consider the authoring and representation of illness narratives in contemporary practice. In particular, I will examine three autobiographical performances: *BALL* by Brian Lobel (2006), *Visiting Hours* by Bob Flanagan (1994) and *RUFF* by Peggy Shaw (2012). The case studies will serve as a focal point for an exploration of strategies within performance that may serve to problematize the status of the patient and provide new perspectives on the medical encounter. The three strategies under discussion are, firstly, re-narrativization, which I identify as a process of creating a performance piece that gives order and a clearly communicable shape to a personal experience of sickness. Secondly, I consider work which may reject a narrativized form and employ a direct encounter with the ill body as a means of challenging dominant cultural understandings of sickness. Finally, I consider pathographic performance as appellation and explore the ways in which a performer may use their experience of suffering as a gateway for connection with the audience.

Pathography

In her seminal text on the subject, Anne Hunsaker Hawkins treats pathography as a subgenre of autobiography. She understands pathography to be a personal narrative that describes experiences of illness and treatment. She notes that this format places the experience of the patient in the centre and that, as such, it is a subjective interpretation of events rather than an historical record. While medical notes will document salient clinical facts, pathography invites the reader/audience to share in a personal exploration of the process of sickness. As a framework for understanding this phenomena, Hunsaker Hawkins draws on sociologist Arthur Frank's notion of the wounded storyteller, an age-old figure whose accounts of her/his own suffering serve as a vehicle of healing – both for themselves and others – re-telling and validating stories and providing a space for valuing and understanding the individual, who may feel isolated by their sickness. Hunsaker Hawkins draws attention to Frank's emphasis on the way in which he says stories are 'told through the body and not about the body' (Frank, in Hunsaker Hawkins, 1999, xvii). I posit that this is particularly true in performance, where the performer's body is in direct relationship with the audience as they give a personal account of their illness experience.

Hunsaker Hawkins is interested in the way in which pathography may concretize the desire to communicate. She describes pathography as 'an artistic product and continuation of the instinctive psychological act of formulation' and, in re-telling the illness narrative, she is interested in how the aesthetic choices that shape the piece are made and how they relate to the psychosomatic experience of sickness (Hunsaker Hawkins, 1999, 24). In this chapter, I will be exploring the particular artistic negotiations which may be related to the creation and presentation of a pathographical performance piece – both in the crafting of text and in the presentation of the body.

Pathography and performance

The most significant element of pathography in performance is the autobiographical staging of the once sick/still sick body. Whereas historical examples of illness dramas were often actors playing out a playwright's perspective on a situation – for example, the exploration of syphilis within Ibsen's *Ghosts* (1882) – pathography marks the direct representation of personal experience. It is possible to suggest that the rise of pathography in performance can be partly attributed to the radical politics of the 1960s and 70s, in particular the second-wave feminist movement, which employed the slogan 'the personal is political'. As Hunsaker Hawkins notes, illness is 'always experienced in relation to a particular configuration of cultural ideologies, practices and attitudes' (1999, 18). For instance, the 'body art' movement of the 1970s onwards can be seen to be an important influence on pathography in performance. In her seminal text on body art, Lea Vergine examines the way in which the artist's own body within such work is used as a 'language' that communicates directly with the audience (2000, 7). The practice of pioneers of body art, such as Gina Pane, whose work explored suffering and pain and often included the presentation of wounds from previous actions, can be understood to be an inspiration to current pathographic artists, as they look to stage elements of their autobiography.

Autobiographical practitioners involved in devising theatre often explicitly draw on their own experience when creating work for performance. This has both methodological and formal implications. Methodologically, the use of personal interests and narratives as source material leads to a complex, reflective, creative process that works around real life data to shape a performance artefact that often combines both truth and fiction. Formally, the presentation of personal material demands a negotiation of the performance of self and appears to invite a particular quality of intimacy from audience members. This is further problematized when working with pathographic material and its embedded cultural baggage. In particular, while other autobiographical performances may deliberately play with the blurring of truth and fiction, pathography often places great emphasis on the authenticity of the material and a performance contract that acknowledges that the performer is sharing an honest account of their illness experiences.

The physical presence of the performer's once/still sick body is the vehicle of communication and serves to substantiate the narrative.

Pathography as re-narrativization

Hunsaker Hawkins notes that pathographies dramatize the sickness events that they describe. She argues that 'Narrative form alters experience, giving it a definite shape, organizing events into a beginning, middle and an end, and adding drama – heightening feelings and seeing the individuals involved as characters in a therapeutic plot' (Hunsaker Hawkins, 1999, 15). Thus, rather than a chaotic, frightening and unpredictable experience, within the pathographic text the period of illness can be understood as a coherent episode, with a clear narrative trajectory. Brian Lobel acknowledges that the process of writing his solo performance piece *BALL* helped to give order and shape to his experience of testicular cancer. In reflecting on the work Lobel says it '[f]elt more like a travelogue that a monologue – I was suddenly a stranger in a strange land and felt compelled to take field notes' (2012a, 13). The piece draws directly on material written during the time Lobel was undergoing and recovering from treatment and the show self-reflexively engages with his negotiation of the sick role. It is overtly autobiographical and unashamedly biased towards his own perspective. As Hunsaker Hawkins notes, whilst a 'medical report disavows any authorship at all (the first person pronoun is almost never used); on the other hand, the authorship of a pathography is never in question' (1999, 13). This is especially true as Lobel is performing his own work and places himself in front of the audience.

Lobel's background in theatre (he was training at the University of Michigan at the time of his diagnosis) suggested his choice to create a performance piece rather than a written narrative but, more than that, Lobel understood solo performance as the 'perfect metaphor for being sick: one body was on stage, isolated and vulnerable just as, when I was hairless, emaciated and sick-looking' (2012a, 14). Lobel saw the work as allowing him to regain a sense of mastery over the illness experience. He said 'Being on the other side of people's often-invasive gaze made me want to take control of such an exchange. Finding a voice and space to speak for oneself'

(2012a, 14). In reflection on the piece, Lobel recognizes the influence of the work of disability scholar Rosemarie Garland-Thomson, who explores the issue of objectification and spectatorship. Garland-Thomson coined the term 'staree' to talk about the experience of being objectified because of disability (2006). Lobel was interested in how staging himself as an object to be stared at and giving overt permission for the gazing to take place might shift the dynamics of the interaction.

Performance scholar Linda Park-Fuller discusses how Lobel is an 'entertainer...one who "stands between" the audience and the world – distracting and diverting it with comedy, but in tragic stories also mediating, guiding or mentoring the audience' (2008, 181). Lobel's structuring of the work enables a safe engagement with others. The piece is crafted according to theatrical convention and punctuated with humour. Lobel assures the audience at the beginning that, although it is a story about cancer, he doesn't die at the end (2012a, 22). The audience recognize that Lobel has recovered and is able to speak to them in the present moment; but there is also a level of anxiety in that the audience are aware that the body that is presented before them has been changed as a result of the interventions described.[1] In performing *BALL*, Lobel is the one mediating the tale, as well as the subject about which the story is told. Literary scholar Louis Renza discusses the split in an autobiographical project between authorial person and authorial persona (quoted in Hunsaker Hawkins, 1999, 16). In Lobel's work this is manifested as the performer appearing in the here and now and presenting what Hunsaker Hawkins terms the 'self-in-crisis' (1999, 17).

Hunsaker Hawkins notes that the liminal quality of a sickness episode can engender questions of identity and place the self in a precarious position. Liminality, as outlined by anthropologist Victor Turner, is a time out of time, set apart from usual social engagement and convention (1995). Hence, when somebody is ill, they step out of their usual social role and enter into a period with different norms – for example, wearing nightclothes during the day and eating special foods. As noted in relation to the figure of the wounded storyteller, it is arguably this status of an outsider that engages others and certainly where pathography is most divergent from the medical narrative in its exploration of the unstable, emotional journey of illness. One section of *BALL* juxtaposes the two forms of narrative explicitly. Lobel gives a detailed description of chemotherapy protocols but intersperses a lyrical account of his physical and emotional reactions to the treatment. Lobel also demonstrates his knowledge of the pathographic form and states: 'In all cancer stories, there is the requisite dark chapter, the hard stuff. I originally wrote *BALL* without one, but because it is a requirement, they made me go back and put it in' (2012a, 38). Lobel employs theatrical devices to display the vulnerability of the body and engage the audience in his subjective experience. For example, his account of the way in which his abdomen was tapped to remove the fluid retention caused by leaking lymph nodes was symbolized by dumping 6.3 litres of water on-stage. This dramatic moment ended the 'dark' section and was immediately punctuated by Lobel's direct address to the audience: 'I'm sorry. I tried to get through that part as quickly as possible!' which reinstated the authorial persona and the safety of the performance frame away from the visceral reality of a body-in-crisis (2012a, 44).

Lobel's self-reflexive work keeps bringing the audience back to the structure of the story. His overt engagement with the form of pathography proves to be a driving force in the narrative. Hunsaker Hawkins discusses the mythic formation of pathography, where cultural belief systems lend metaphorical shape to the expectations and experience of illness. In particular, she notes models, such as the 'athletic paradigm', which encompasses the idea that the ill person should be an 'achiever', with an obligation to undertake publicly some feat of courage or endurance (1999, 76). Lobel plays with this notion within his piece. He employs the conceit of comparing his own appearance, struggle and achievements to that of world class athlete Lance Armstrong who famously documented his return to sporting life after testicular cancer. Lobel states within the piece 'I need to be a hero. A role model. A SURVIVOR! ... You can't just survive cancer anymore' (2012a, 48). With humorous effect, Lobel describes how his quest to be a hero led him to the Hospital Stem Cell Transplant Reunion Picnic Hula Hoop Contest. While hula-ing in front of the audience he speaks of the 'pressure of Lance Armstrong-like success' and his determination to beat an eight-year-old girl in the competition; along with the devastation of the moment when his hula-hoop fell (2012a, 51). He recognizes that this incident undercuts the narrative expectation of victory and states: 'That wasn't supposed to happen. I was supposed to be victorious. I was supposed to learn to love myself and to learn that winning doesn't matter, and then I was supposed to win anyway' (2012a, 52). The bathetic ending, where Lobel wins by default, as his eight-year-old competitor is disqualified, serves to highlight the pervasiveness of the hero narrative as a means of providing a satisfactory closure.

On reflection, Lobel was unhappy with the narrative of events he presented in *BALL*. He states: 'BALL was a survivor story … [it] attempted to highlight the clichés of "the cancer story" while engaging in every single one' (2012a, 15). As a writer, he was aware of the acceptable conventions of illness drama and became uncomfortable in the material that he had edited out in trying to construct his hero narrative. He states: 'I wanted to start talking about the filthy stories, the inappropriate stories, that coincide with having cancer in your genitals' (1999, 15). He felt the need to write another show – *Other Funny Stories About Cancer* – in which he included the self-censored material. As might be expected for a piece that is not so narratively driven (in terms of creating a good story), it was less formally structured and finished with Lobel stating: 'And I guess that's an ending' (2012a, 78). It is interesting to read performance scholar John T. Warren's response to a performance of *BALL*. Even though Lobel explicitly states within the piece 'I want not to learn from this' (2012a, 33) Warren asserts that it 'is as if he offers us a moral: … I have lessons to offer from my experiences' (2008, 185). This seems to affirm the ubiquity of the cultural expectation for an improving experience when witnessing pathographical performance.

Pathography as cultural intervention

In developing *Other Funny Stories About Cancer*, Lobel drew inspiration from the work of Bob Flanagan. Flanagan suffered from cystic fibrosis, a hereditary disease that affects the glands and lungs and makes breathing and digestion particularly difficult. Before his death in 1996, Flanagan spent a lot of his life in hospital and his experience of his own ill body shaped his life and work. As a person with a life-limiting disease, Flanagan embraced working with the body in crisis and was explicit about how his masochistic practice sought to explore his pain threshold and control the discomfort that he experienced on a daily basis due to his illness. Flanagan engaged in extreme actions, such as hammering nails through his genitals.[2] Rather than the narrative reconstruction offered by Lobel, the focus of Flanagan's work is the body as object and he clearly works within the realm of body art. Without narrative framing there is direct contact with the sick body and Vergine explores how work which engages with the 'real' in this way may serve to destroy the artificial screen that separates the public from the private (2000, 16). So Flanagan presents his own body and private activities, such as the sado-masochistic acts performed with Sheree Rose (his long-term partner and collaborator) within the public realm and offers this as an intervention into how the sick body is represented and understood.

Literary scholar Linda Kauffman describes Flanagan's work as 'Sadomedicine' in that it 'fuses medicine with sadomasochism to problematize the relationships between the social and the psychic, between disease and desire' (1998a, 31). The conventional conception of the illness experience is that the sick person is expected to passively submit to the superior knowledge of clinicians who will objectively examine and treat their bodies. Flanagan's work can be seen to play with this role of patient. He is compliant, in fact his masochism plays compliance in an excessive manner, yet he is also difficult in that he refuses to contain his suffering to the niche allotted to him. An illustrative example of this work is *Visiting Hours*, a site-related installation made jointly with Sheree Rose.[3]

Visiting Hours transformed the art space into a hospital ward which was complete with waiting room, medical X-rays and, at the heart of the piece, the ill body of Bob Flanagan himself, in a hospital bed. The exhibition catalogue for the New Museum states: 'The installation is designed like a crazy stage set of a children's residential hospital, replete with torture chamber lurking amongst the institutional cheer' (1994). There were child-like elements within the work – such as wooden building blocks juxtaposing the letters CF and SM – alongside more explicitly sexualized objects, for example, a medical stool with a butt plug glued to the seat. The transformation of medical tools into sexual equipment is troubling in that it can be seen to force the spectator to think about the corporeal reality and sexuality of diseased bodies – material that Lobel edited out of *BALL*. In presenting this material Flanagan can be seen to invite cultural reflection and self-consciously questions the position of the ill person. Barilan notes that Flanagan's performances refuse to accept the standards of normality and a 'tyranny of health' and his work self-reflexively sets up a discussion of what it means to be perceived as 'sick' (2004, 11). Indeed, Flanagan's stated agenda was to 'fight sickness with sickness' (quoted in Kauffman, 1998a, 21). In placing this work in the public realm, Flanagan's body becomes a site/sight for public debate and a re-negotiation of clinical discourse. His art can be seen as an intervention in cultural understandings of illness that places the patient as passive and helpless, and dependent on the professional help of others. *Visiting Hours* turned spectators into active participants as they negotiated the medical scene promenade-style. Unlike a conventional hospital environment, visitors were encouraged to interact with the equipment and images and were invited to see them as props that stage the sick body, as well as reflecting on how agents of healing may actually inflict pain. Within the event, Flanagan, the patient, took an active role, returning the gaze of the audience and confronting visitors with their own voyeurism. It appears that the spectators were aware of Flanagan's position as witness and, to his surprise, drew him in as confessor to their whispered stories by his bedside. Kauffman notes how *Visiting Hours* performed the traditional role of pathography in that it was charting unmapped territory through presenting the audience with an experience of terminal illness and a medicalized setting. She states: 'We know we must die, but the knowledge remains theoretical until "the end"' (1998b, 38). The corporeal reality of Flanagan's installation invited the audience to engage in direct negotiation with the unknown.

In a critique of pathographic writing, journalist Decca Aitkenhead, in *The Guardian*, posits that the relationship between reader and writer is sentimental and easily abandoned because readers are only 'consumers' of intimacy, rather than engaging in a meaningful relationship (1999, 15). As I have noted, pathographical performance offers a different experience to the written form in that the audience are engaged in a live encounter with the subject of the material and, I would suggest, works against sentimentality and the superficial connection that Aitkenhead suggests. Lobel appears to resist sentimentality through the use of humour and Flanagan through excessive and explicit representation. Kauffman states: 'Sentimentality is the death of feeling, and all of Flanagan's art is about living with heightened feeling, sensation, consciousness'

(1998a, 34). Flanagan invites spectators to observe the messiness of sickness that exceeds the sanitized illness dramas played out on mainstream television. Although different in strategy, like Lobel, Flanagan's work can be seen to open up a discursive space for the exploration of fears and fantasies and alternative ways of being with illness. He uses his performance work as a cultural intervention to challenge received notions and offer alternatives.

Pathography as appellation

Hunsaker Hawkins suggests that pathography offers an effective vehicle of expression in that it acts as a means to link the self, which is suffering, with the wider world. This follows on from Frank's notion that, while disease may set a body apart, the wounded storyteller's story serves to connect them to others through 'the common bond of suffering that joins bodies in their shared vulnerability' (1995, xi). As literary scholar Harold Schweitzer notes, pain can be understood as an isolating experience. Yet Schweitzer argues that, while pain is addressed to no-one, suffering (the outward expression of an individual's pain) is 'always an appellation of the other' (2002) – drawing on the French word *appeler*, that is to call. In this final example, I shall explore how pathographical performance may 'call' to the audience.

RUFF, co-written and performed by Peggy Shaw, draws on her experience of stroke in 2011.[4] Shaw is an accomplished performer with a long history of using autobiographical material in performance to address socio-political issues – particularly through her work with Split Britches.[5] More recently, Shaw has been developing solo pieces such as *The Menopausal Gentleman* (1998) and *Must: The Inside Story* (2007) that have reflected upon her ageing body.[6] As with her other shows, the speaking body within *RUFF* is the site of performance and provides both the impetus for and the means to communicate. Shaw sees artistic production as an opportunity to 'fill up the spaces in my brain' that have been left by the stroke (2014). Within the piece, the stroke becomes artistic material – the title refers to the three stroke ruff which is recommended to Shaw as a place to begin when learning to play the drums. The piece is carefully woven together from fragmented elements that reflect Shaw's experience of life after the trauma.

Shaw takes an aesthetic perspective on illness and describes stroke as 'a deadly finger of ice', as a means to communicate the essence of the experience to her audience (2014). In exploring the incommunicability of a painful experience, literary scholar Elaine Scarry observes that, when describing pain, a person may couch their description within metaphor. So they may say 'It feels like a knife' (1985, 16). This description does not exactly match the feelings of pain but it serves to externalize it and thus 'make shareable' the experience. I would argue, however, that such a description does not serve to objectify the pain in the manner which Scarry describes but, instead, serves to subjectify it, that is to say that the person who is listening to the description comes to an understanding through an imaginative encounter with their own body. I would argue that, in the attempt to communicate, the expression of pain asks for a response from the listener and that response demands an awareness of their own body. Pathographic performance raises awareness of shared vulnerability. Like Lobel, who has a section within *BALL* which encourages the audience to carry out a testicle/breast exam, Shaw counsels her audience to remember FAST – the acronym reminding of the signs of stroke – and asking the audience to turn and assess each other invites an awareness that this could easily happen to any of them. At the beginning of the piece she invites participation, asking audience members to hold items for her that she uses during the show.

In his review of *RUFF*, Benjamin Gillespie focuses on the sense of vulnerability of the performer and the awareness of the way in which the trauma has impacted upon the body presented to the audience (2013). The performance is an exploration of embodied knowledge and a demonstration of the corporeal effects of the condition. Critic Taffy Jaffe's account of the piece states that Shaw '[d]oesn't just tell us, she shows us' (2014). The members of the audience are witness to Shaw's attempt to resume function post-stroke and the accommodations that are needed for her new state of being. The damage to her brain means that Shaw cannot remember all the lines and so monitors are needed to prompt her within the performance. These are placed in the centre of the performance space and become an integral part of the piece – sometimes displaying images that Shaw is describing to the audience; sometimes turned away; and sometimes providing a form of sub-title as the screens display the script as written, which juxtapose with the text as

Shaw is remembering it in the moment. The latter element serves to heighten the awareness of the 'here-and-now' of the performance event, where the audience are witness to the self-exposure of the pathographic subject. Shaw gives a subjective account of her illness. She offers alternative reasons to those of the clinicians as to why her stroke may have occurred: she suggests that it was caused by a friend, who had recently died, wanting to take Shaw with her to the other side. There is also more explicit critique within the text of the medical treatment Shaw received – from a story of a brusque nurse who shook her awake to ask if she wanted a sleeping tablet; to the assertion that after the stroke she felt the comforting presence of her deceased sister Norma living inside her but that the treatment had 'removed [Norma] perfectly' and left Shaw feeling empty (2014). Shaw asserts that, although an MRI scan is able to provide a picture of her brain, it can't photograph her thoughts. It seems that this thought process is what *RUFF* attempts to give a demonstration of, and in so doing, invites recognition of the subjective processes of memory, loss and love that lie beneath a medical trauma.

Conclusion

Whilst this chapter has explored three very different pieces which, in themselves, indicate the idiosyncrasy of illness and its interpretation by artists, I would suggest that there are some common themes and tactics to be identified within their working practices. In their survey of theatre, therapy and public health, performance scholars Jill MacDougall and P. Stanley Yoder suggest that there is a fundamental difference in the way in which artists approach sickness. They state: 'Artists respond to the afflictions of the collective body ... by directly addressing the social context and creating public forums to seek solutions, whereas physicians tend to pull back into biotechnology and to medicalize social problems' (1998, 2). In all the pieces explored in this chapter, the public and direct negotiation has been particularly significant, as the artists literally put their bodies on the line in front of a live audience. Although their pathographic work may offer a critique of clinical practice, the artists under discussion here have not been in direct opposition to medicine – indeed Flanagan's doctors, in particular, can be seen as collaborators in his work, co-operating with filming and visiting his exhibitions – but the artists have offered a unique outlook on the patient experience from the standpoint of those undergoing/having undergone treatment. In pathographic performance, the artists are active curators of their own story, working self-consciously and self-reflexively to offer an insight into happenings which are often hidden from public view. Through the strategies of re-narrativization, cultural intervention and appellation, the performance work discussed in this chapter serves to open up discursive space for exploring alternative ways of being with illness. They re-frame cultural narratives and issue a call to the audience to engage in an exploration of suffering and a shared sense of vulnerability. Whilst this is not the athletic paradigm, it is certainly an act of courage and endurance.

6

Fun with Cancer Patients: The Affect of Cancer

Brian Lobel

Picture your life after cancer

In April 2010, *The New York Times Online* published 'Picture Your Life After Cancer', a user-generated photo essay collecting stories and images from cancer survivors. 'For the estimated twelve million cancer survivors in the United States', the feature begins, 'some of life's biggest challenges begin after the treatment ends' (Barrow and Jackson, 2010). Although the feature recognizes difficult consequences of illness, its focus is clearly centred on positive outcomes, asserting that 'the cancer experience can lead to a shift in priorities, bring new insights or work as a catalyst to quit a job or try something new' (2010). The photographs deliver accordingly, with images of the Eiffel Tower, snow peaked mountains and cycling races dominating the landscape.

Accompanying the photo essay, readers are able to submit comments, most of which are devoted to individuals promoting their cancer blogs or expanding on the information in their photo submission. Inside these margins – perhaps tellingly 'inside the margins' – a singular voice challenges the presumptions of 'Picture Your Life' in a striking manner. In the pithiest response to the article, a woman identifying herself only as 'Claire' writes 'Cancer ruined my fetility [*sic*] and my sex life. I was twenty-six when diagnosed. Life sucks now. Not what you were looking for?' (Parker-Pop, 2010). Claire's sentence rips through the photo essay and the bodies it features, which are healthy, fit and full of positivity. The statement draws attention to the un-photographable nature of her experience and alerts a reader to ask how a photograph of infertility or a ruined sex life looks. And if a photograph of this body, which is not healthy, fit or full of positivity were taken, would *The New York Times Online* allow it to be published?

Claire's question is rhetorical, based on her knowledge of how positive messages around cancer are policed. Although her question presumes an individual experience, Claire's singular voice is joined by a small chorus of commentators using her as a springboard for sharing. The formulaic nature of 'Picture Your Life After Cancer' seems to expect a certain type of response from its readership, tapping into the cult of positivity which is particular to public discussions of cancer treatment and cancer survivorship (discussed by Barbara Ehrenreich in *Bright-Sided*, 2009) and making limited space for alternative tones around cancer treatment or survivorship. More importantly, however, these projects limit what is really known about bodies with cancer, these bodies which are so often discussed but so often misunderstood.

Fun with cancer patients

The goal of my performance practice for over ten years has been to create space for alternative and truthful narratives around illness that promote reflection on how cancer is discussed, framed and read by audiences, particularly from voices which have been marginalized by either their content or their tone. In this chapter, I will examine two pieces that were created as part of *Fun with Cancer Patients* (FWCP), a project that was developed through two Wellcome Trust Arts Awards (2010 and 2013) and created in collaboration with Birmingham Teenage Cancer Trust at Fierce Festival in 2013. FWCP is an on-going exhibition project dedicated to raising the intellectual understanding of the cancer experience and, particularly, the experience of bodies with cancer. By taking as its subject the embodied reality of cancer – the smells, the annoyances, the pleasures, the absurdities – FWCP explores the psychosocial aspects of illness and provides patient participants with an opportunity to reflect on their unique embodied experience – and the wisdom that has derived from this reflection.

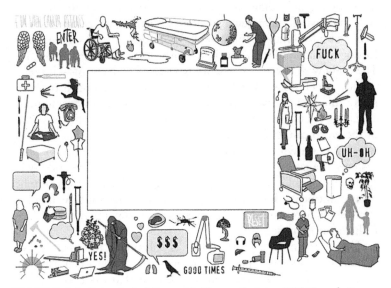

FIGURE 6.1 *Brian Lobel,* Fun with Cancer Patients *(2013): website.*

This chapter uses two 'Actions' from FWCP to illustrate how the embodied experience of cancer might be explored through performance – defined here as any live artistic action done for an audience of any size – in ways that free patients from cultural expectations of cancer survivorship. Drawn from interventionist methodologies and examples, the Guerilla Pub Quiz offers an unexpected representation of a cancer survivor, one that complicates the 'burden of representation' and that exposes the unknowability of cancer experience. The private Action of Yoga at St Barts ('performed' only for an exhibition audience who witnessed its documentation) raises the question of who such performances are for, complicating issues around the intended effects and affects of performance. In both cases, the one-off Action is presented to audiences through their documentation so that it is primarily the documentation, presented at the exhibition, rather than the Action, which 'performs'.

The body with cancer is an unknown body, and a body that is essentially unknowable to anyone else, including an individual before their own cancer diagnosis. Lyotard's differend, or 'the unstable state and instant of language wherein something which must be able to be put into phrases cannot yet be' provides a useful starting point for the unknowability of the body with cancer (Lyotard, 1988, 13). The body with cancer – particularly soon after diagnosis – becomes a body which does not quite understand itself. Although there are many things that disturb a body's constitution and understanding of itself – ageing, accidents, violence, other diseases – the heaviness of the word cancer (and its position as something within the body which has grown malignantly and unnoticed by the body's usual systems) causes a radical shift. And given that the body with cancer is a public body – diagnosis is often marked by a number of appointments, histories being taken, 'comings out' to families/friends/employers – there is an even greater imperative to put these feelings into phrases.

This relearning of the body is captured in crisp artistic language by photographer Jo Spence, who upon diagnosis with breast cancer, wrote 'I realised with horror that my body was not made of photographic paper, nor was it an image, or an idea, or a psychic structure [...] it was made of blood, bones and tissue. Some of them now appeared to be cancerous' (Spence, 1986, 151). If Spence previously conceived of her body as a stable image or psychic structure able to be photographed, it appears that diagnosis demonstrated that artistic metaphor – even for an artist with a personally and politically-invested methodology – necessarily made way for bodily reality, post-diagnosis. And just as Lyotard discussed the urgency of finding phrases with the differend, the pressure for Spence to find these new 'phrases' (or artistic methodologies) forced new partnerships and new approaches to art-making.

Despite the intensity of the experience of diagnosis, and the medical and personal resources that seem to snap into high gear when an individual is diagnosed, the language around cancer still reeks with simple representations: either large-scale fundraising campaigns or inspirational tomes, none of which actually speak to cancer patients of the physical, emotional and/or psychological realities they are facing. Without any accurate representations or public conversation about the what, how and why of cancer, the body with cancer remains unknowable. FWCP queries bodies with cancer not only to make these bodies knowable to the broader public (thus injecting discourses with new information and new angles) but, most importantly, FWCP provides opportunities for the patient participants to make their bodies known to themselves, in whatever tone or format of documentation is appropriate and desired.

The process is simple: I work with a specific individual or group of patient participants to discuss what they want or need – in relation to their illness – and then work with them to create an extravagant Action to address this want or need. Previous Actions have included pop-up kitchens and far-flung car trips. Actions are then documented and displayed alongside critical reflections from patients and medical advisors on subjects such as post-treatment anxiety, the language of illness, the development/ loss of friendships, hair loss, decrease/increase of appetite and beyond.

I hope to demonstrate that FWCP may provide a space of engagement for those who find the tools established for the public exhibition of bodies with cancer (and bodies with histories of cancer) to be limiting and reaffirming of a policed positivity. I argue that the project opens up new spaces for expression to capture a patient-focused experience inside of performance creation and reception. By denying an audience an immediate interaction with – or story from – a body with cancer, and particularly with the smiling, fit bodies they are accustomed to seeing on advertisements for cancer fundraisers or inspirational stories, FWCP also engages with audience members' distance from a one-off performance Action (instead being witness only to its documentation), as a metaphor for understanding embodied experience.

Eat me: Research, development and canvases

By refusing to tell the story of a person with cancer from start to finish, FWCP avoids the dichotomy of Survivorship Story or Bereavement Story, which, as Jackie Stacey suggests, frames most cancer narratives (Stacey, 1997, 2). The performance and documentation process for all of the FWCP Actions derives from a reflection on the work of Hayley Newman, and in particular in her work *Connotations: Performance Images 1994–1998* (1998). The work, a series of photographs and accompanying texts taken from a fictional series of one-off performance events, highlights the tension between a performed action and its documentation and was, for Newman, a reflection on 'the experience of performing and its archiving as a document' (Newman, 2004, 166). What Newman does so effectively in *Connotations* is to blur or challenge the line between 'truth' and 'fiction' and 'real-life' experience and performance. Although the Actions in FWCP (described below) were very much real events, made by people affected by malignancies, the process of creating and documenting the Actions inherently blurs the line between truth and fiction. The private nature of these events and the subjectivity encouraged by documentation (which will be the only object available for public consumption) makes the borders between who is affected and who is not affected by cancer more porous – a useful place for FWCP to encourage its viewership to be when developing a more inclusive cancer conversation.

FWCP contained the explicit goal of creating ten different art objects, (documenting ten different Actions) which would be exhibited at the Mac Birmingham in the UK, exploring ten different psychosocial realities of cancer. The project sought to use live art methodologies to create discreet, one-off Actions that would offer new perspectives on the cancer experience. These individual perspectives could then be put together and, as a group, allow a complex, potentially conflicting experience for public audiences.

The tension between involving participants in a project, which is mostly centred on the increased learning of a 'general public' (unseen by participants creating Actions), brought significant challenges and it was ethical considerations which inspired the FWCP interactive Canvas, first created as a recruiting tool and later updated and exhibited as a hands-on exhibition piece. Graphic designer Nako Okubo, computer designer Chipp Jansen and I created a small activity that was capable of being both serious and playful in equal measure. The Canvas function consists of over 100 images, each based on a particular item from either cancer treatment or the embodied experience of illness. The images were derived from my own history and from cancer blogs and existing narratives. Traditional medical imagery such as X-ray machines, gurneys and nurses are mixed on the palette with images less-commonly displayed in relation to cancer, such as bed pans, amputated arms, vomit and marijuana.

Responding to imagery like that inside 'Picture Your Life', a stark black-and-white motif was chosen which, although playful, felt radically different from the colourful, yellow-ribbon-dotted pictures. Images were made malleable through a simple computer programme that allowed each image to be independently resized and repositioned. This simple tool allowed for a myriad of stories to be told and a number of embodied experiences to be represented. While pictures of cancer bodies are treated with a policed positivity, these black and white outlines of bodies can be flipped, stabbed and maltreated in ways which might be adequate metaphors for the cancer experience.

Upon seeing the Canvas depicted in Figure 6.2 during the research and development stage, I hoped that its creator would want to collaborate on an Action. Something about the Canvas' gallows humour – an image of a skull being prodded by a fork, a knife and even a tea bag – struck me as funny and provocative. The image, for me, encapsulated the disempowering feeling of having your body prodded and poked by nurses, doctors and medical students. The accompanying text of simply 'Eat Me', however, pushed through the imagery in a manner similar to Claire's response to 'Picture Your Life' in that it was bold, personal and undocument-able. The body, which actually experienced the shuffling and prodding, and which could never be meaningfully photographed, could here be represented metaphorically and presented (not as a body but as a set of ideas) for honest public dialogue. When Laura, the Canvas' creator, emailed a few minutes later with an idea for an Action, our collaboration began.

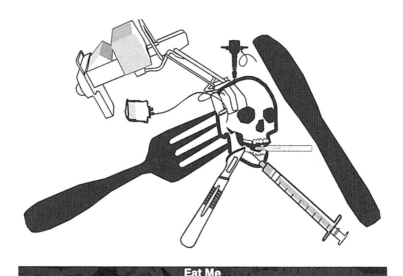

Eat Me

FIGURE 6.2 *Brian Lobel,* Fun with Cancer Patients (2013): *Laura's submission to the interactive canvas.*

In this chapter, I will consider two of the three Actions created with Laura as part of the research and development process (the other eight Actions are available on the online archive). I have chosen to reflect on the two created with Laura as they most directly reference the body with cancer, and particularly the known/unknown body. The two Actions I will analyse, Yoga at St Barts and Guerilla Pub Quiz, most succinctly highlight the effort to challenge how traditional cancer narratives play with iconography and demonstrate how the process may open up new ways of seeing and engaging with bodies with cancer.

Yoga at St Barts

For Laura, one of the most powerful, embodied experiences of post-cancer living was the nausea and anxiety that she would experience when leaving St Paul's tube station in London and walking towards the hospital:

I'd make that journey every time I had chemotherapy, knowing that I'd come to the hospital, be pumped full of drugs and leave feeling awful. So I'd start to feel sick even before I'd arrive at the hospital. There are little triggers along the way, the smell of the Café Nero, the smell of the coffee shop here, and the sound of the builders. All of these things helped trigger 'Oh I'm going to the hospital. I'm going to feel really ill for the next few weeks.' (in Lobel et al., 2013)

As we reflected on this experience – an experience which I had not shared – the answer to the question 'What would you do that would be helpful?' always seemed to return to the hospital, and transforming it in some way. Yoga at St Barts developed nearly instantly and organically: a sunrise yoga session in the middle of St Bartholomew's Hospital, for just Laura and an instructor. 'The idea with the Action', Laura stated, 'is to make the hospital a safe place, a happy place' (Lobel et al., 2013).

In order to contextualize each Action into a conversation about cancer experience, the documentation of the Actions were discussed with Sue Gessler, a clinical psychologist working in gynaecological cancers. Gessler's expertise was pursued to probe whether each Action represented a rare experience with cancer, or if other patients experienced the same realities. Gessler was asked to add professional context: Why do patients pursue activities such as yoga? Is it purely relaxation or is there something more at play? Gessler writes:

Yoga is about working the body, you're breaking down the stance between mind and body. The body with cancer can become hated – patients will say 'I can't think about this part of my body' or 'I don't think from here down'. Yoga is actually reconnecting people with their body in a more neutral way. (in Lobel et al., 2013)

Yoga at St Barts effectively highlighted the desire for calm, and a process by which post-treatment anxiety and discomfort with the body post-cancer can be addressed directly (even if for a day).

Gessler explained the Action without analysing the 'state' of the participants. It felt essential that Laura's Action be developed without pre-emption from a psychological professional, shielding Laura from what might be perceived as an overpowering medical system or policed positivity determining how her body needed to experience her cancer. With this process, the Action remained a yoga class between Laura, Angelika, Olga (who documented the work via twenty drawings in a sketchbook) and myself (audio recording the event). At no point was Laura asked to celebrate her survivorship or bemoan her body; she was not asked how effective this day of yoga was in reshaping her post-treatment anxiety. Instead, the Action allowed Laura to participate in something that fulfilled a particular need, while the performance for exhibition audiences (later looking at the drawings and hearing Angelika's yoga instruction) provided an opportunity to reflect on how chemotherapy may leave indelible embodied memories.

The creating of distance for the audience is a conscious effort: not only does documentation remind the audience that they were not at the yoga class, but it also reminds them they are not necessarily privy to the emotional secrets of a person with cancer. Using twenty sketches and an audio recording as the documentation reinforced this distancing in that audience members could not always track the audio, requiring them to piece together the event themselves. The piece never claims to be Laura's full story, but rather an attempt to intervene in her anxiety.

The Action's privacy also demonstrates that FWCP does not propose to 'help anyone' directly, except those present. Although there is strength in community, there is something equally powerful in knowing that your life does not need to inspire others. In this way, FWCP achieves Arthur W. Frank's goal stated in *The Wounded Storyteller* of shifting the 'dominant cultural conception of illness away from passivity – the ill person as "victim of" disease and then recipient of care – toward activity' (Frank, 1995, xi). I argue that FWCP goes even farther than Frank's suggestion by putting Laura's Action in dialogue with Thompson's idea of non-effect.

In *Performance Affects*, Thompson asks 'How do we make work that is permitted not to promise effect?' (2009, 183). If the explicit goal of FWCP was effect, then the documentation of the work or its public iteration would demonstrate how much the various groups of participants learned, received or grew as a part of the Action-making process. Instead, it was FWCP's affect on the exhibition audience that was the goal of the project, awakening, as Thompson writes, 'individuals to possibilities beyond themselves without an insistence on what the experience is – what meanings should be attached' (2009, 111). Because Laura was not asked to have her yoga class teach or do anything, Yoga at St Barts – as an Action she created – empowered a truly active moment which, seemingly-ironically, effected nothing.

Guerilla Pub Quiz

The Guerilla Pub Quiz did not take the body of cancer patients as its central focus – instead focusing on the more internal phenomenon of 'chemo brain' – but featured a bold and (for audiences that were inside the pub and who later watch the documentation) uncomfortable presentation of a very empowered cancer body, one which was brash and outspoken, scarred and visible. In our preparatory conversations, Laura had talked extensively about memory loss or 'chemo brain' and questioned whether it was a real thing, or a convenient excuse for inattention. The answer, therefore, to FWCP's question 'What would you do that would be helpful?' became 'I would celebrate my memory loss'. And celebrate she did, with Guerilla Pub Quiz which was staged as an intervention at Off-Broadway in Hackney, London, with questions relating to Laura's cancer. By crafting a competition in which competitors who answer the most questions incorrectly win, Laura flipped the expectation that to have memory loss is tragic. Guerilla Pub Quiz featured Laura's stand-up persona, presenting material without reverential hush and, recognizing the usual severity around cancer, even provided an opportunity for audience members to rename cancer. 'Last year', she announced 'I was diagnosed with kittens'. The Action, however, did not shy away from difficult territory, covering her presumed chances of survival, of recurrence and asking how many women were diagnosed with breast cancer in Britain each day.

Amidst a relatively fast-paced interaction with her audience, the question that caused the most commotion (to borrow usage from Sandahl and Auslander to describe the commotion caused by disabled bodies in public space (2005, 2)) was a question very few polite acquaintances would ask: 'Which one of my boobs is fake, left or right?' It was a complex question as it was said so proudly that the audience almost forgot that this was her body put forward for examination, her body with scars, with surgeries. Her body which is forever negotiating its 'realness' or 'fakeness' in front of strangers. While there are significant projects (particularly photography projects) which have taken on mastectomy scars as their subject, the appearance of bodies with breast cancer are still quite rare, and Laura here negotiated it powerfully. After asking this particular question, Laura invited the stare – and audience members instantly asked her to shake her chest. While she initially conceded and shook, she quickly relented, 'That gives it away', she said.

The intense 'visual engagement' of a stare, Garland-Thomson writes, 'creates a circuit of communication and meaning-making. Staring bespeaks involvement, and being stared at demands a response. A staring encounter is a dynamic struggle – starers inquire, starees lock eyes or flee, and starers advance or retreat: one moves forward and the other moves back' (Garland-Thomson, 2009, 2–3). By recognizing the give and take of the stare, Garland-Thomson opens up the potential for pleasure and equity (or if not absolute equity, some sort of parity) in the relationship. The existence of pleasure and equity marks quite a progressive step forward from the pervasive rubric of 'the gaze', which sees the relationship between starer and staree as inherently oppressive (Garland-Thomson, 2009, 10). While audience members were seemingly staring at Laura's body in this moment, it is clear that the entirety of the question was a strategy for her to engage that stare – and to stare directly back.

The public nature of Guerilla Pub Quiz, as different to Yoga at St Barts, was perhaps its most notable feature and the overwhelming majority of those in the pub were not aware that any event would be taking place. Guerilla Pub Quiz succeeded in bringing cancer (and a proud cancer body) to a space that is imagined to be cancer-free, in hopes of integrating cancer into everyday conversation. This integration is an imperative mission, but not always a painless process, and in a handful of cases, audience members at the pub were quite unnerved by the performance.

The reflections on the Guerilla Pub Quiz by Gessler allows the pub quiz to speak to larger issues related to cancer while, again, freeing Laura from carrying the 'burden of representation' (Morley and Chen, 1996, 442). Gessler begins by drawing attention to why 'chemo brain' is such a misunderstood or under-researched phenomenon: 'Chemo brain is really, really interesting because there's been a long history of patients complaining about it and people rather ignoring it because it's not 'sinister'. Everything to do with cancer is ignored if it's not about the illness itself' (in Lobel et al., 2013).

Identifying the biases inside the medical profession helps the viewer of the documentation think critically about medicine and understand it as a subjective process, affected by funding priorities and cultural context. If the previous goal of oncologists was to keep patients alive at any cost, a phenomenon like 'chemo brain' may not be a priority of cancer research.

But chemo brain, if not a scientific fact, is a current part of cancer conversation. A statement from University College London Hospital's Head Nurse, Anne Lanceley, elucidates this point, explaining that the term chemo brain is 'generated by people with cancer talking to each other. It's a cancer-sufferers or – survivors' terminology which is not a medical language. It seems empowering that it comes from the grassroots and not that it originates from a doctor' (in Lobel et al., 2013). The 'grassroots nature' of the chemo brain conversation frames Laura's Action by positioning Laura's experience as one of many, redressing the absence of concrete scientific answers to this phenomenon. Laura takes memory loss as a given, and seemingly does not care whether it is real.

By adding the contextualizing statements after the Action – and without Laura's participation in creating them – the Actions feel like Actions. While the documentation and statements allow the research of FWCP to come to the fore, they do so only in the hope of reducing the pressure placed on the event itself. The pressure for cancer patients and advocates to create something useful or effective (which may be derived from a culture that looks to pity people with cancer and stare at their bodies, thus separating them out as different) remains very real indeed. The mixture of Action, documentation and reflection allowed FWCP to respond to individual desires, outside pressures and, perhaps, the individual desires to appease those outside pressures.

Fun with reflections

Reflecting on Yoga at St Barts, Guerilla Pub Quiz and the entire exhibition in Birmingham makes me feel both confident and unsure about my conclusions, in equal measure. While I am enthusiastic about the final documentation created from the Actions, I am wary about drawing definitive conclusions from the work, or at least too many of them. The Actions and FWCP itself were developed from personal experiences, reacting to what I had experienced and heard in conversation with Laura, as opposed to an extensively researched biomedical or psycho-oncological process. While my reading on cancer and participation in conferences over the years has highlighted for me the importance of thinking about 'chemo brain', the importance of yoga, support systems and the like, there was (and is) no checklist of 'Psychosocial Aspects of Cancer Experience' that needs to be addressed by FWCP. And yet, from a critical perspective, it feels as though the engagement enacted through FWCP comes as a direct result of reading and consideration of practitioners and theorists like Garland-Thomson and Thompson. I believe that the affect created for Laura, audiences to the documentation, the FWCP team and for me is demonstrative of what a conscious research practice might look like. Even this uncertainty, this celebration of the end of effect feels like an appropriate and accurate result.

In January 2011, *The Guardian Weekend* featured a cover story entitled 'Cancer: the new normal' with an image of a supermarket filled with bald customers. The article (an excerpt from Siddhartha Mukherjee's *The Emperor of All Maladies* (2011b)) puts forward the provocative idea that cancer is a normal process, and describes how the disease is 'stitched into our genetic being' (Mukherjee, 2011a, 23). 'The question', Mukherjee continues, 'then will not be if we will encounter this immortal illness in our lives, but when'. Such a statement does not fly in the face of cancer research efforts or advocacy campaigns focused at curbing exposure to known carcinogens, but does sit in stark opposition to features like 'Picture Your Life After Cancer', with its strong bias towards positive changes post-cancer. While these efforts may mean to inspire survivors or promote funding for research, they also increase a separation of the cancer experience – and bodies with cancer – from the everyday. Even if a 'cure' for cancer (an incredibly reductive term considering the ways in which cancer functions) is found in our generation, if the focus is only on survivorship and cure, cure, cure, so much of the messy, ambiguous, difficult embodied experiences may remain unspoken about and unspoken for. These unknown bodies – the focus of so much public attention – will remain forever so in their medical, psychosocial or emotional dimensions. Although FWCP does not use performance methodologies to cure malignant growth or to effect particular medical changes, it does attempt to impact the overall affect of cancer, to curb the very real pressures that keep those with cancer from seeing honest representations of their lived experiences and their bodies, bodies which remain a flashpoint for both public fascination and repulsion.

7

DOC: The Narrative Performance of Expertise

P. Solomon Lennox and Fiona Pettit

The DOC: An overview

The term diabetes online community (DOC) refers to a multifarious network of social media outlets, primarily concerned with providing connection and community for people with diabetes (PWD). The DOC incorporates, but is not limited to, blogs and micro-blogging platforms and makes use of still and moving images, audio and text to engage with, portray and perform the narrative identities of individuals associated with diabetes. Whilst the community is primarily run by and for PWD, the community also represents and connects with medical professionals, representatives from pharmaceutical companies, local and national governments and individuals who do not have diabetes but live with someone who does.

The community provides a space where the medical, commercial, popular and public narratives of diabetes, illness, and management interact with the personal auto-ethnographic accounts of PWD. This interaction is important, particularly when exploring notions of objecthood and subjecthood within the performance of science.

This chapter explores how PWD engage with performative practices in order to navigate and perform narratives of diabetes. These narratives incorporate terms such as *care*, *compliance* and *management* and, in doing so, navigate the complex relationship between diverse knowledge systems. The DOC offers a degree of diversity in terms of the types of narratives performed and, as such, the type of expertise exhibited, owned and performed online.

By adopting Arthur Frank's typology of bodies, this chapter demonstrates that the DOC provides a space where PWD can perform and interact with notions of the *disciplined body* through *self-regimentation* and narratives and actions concerned with control (Frank, 1995, 41). However, unlike previous coverage of the DOC (see Silverman, 2012), this chapter is not concerned with how social media platforms facilitate better control of diabetes, the extent to which they promote compliance with medical procedures and expertise, or the manner in which PWD are able to demonstrate improved management of their chronic illness. Rather, this chapter explores how the performative practices exhibited in the DOC enable PWD to explore and expand upon narratives of the disciplined body, to offer new stories of subjecthood from the perspective of the expert patient.

From PWD as objects to PWD as subjects

Foucault asserts that human beings began to be considered as scientific objects in the nineteenth century (Foucault, 1970, 376). Languages developed to articulate the knowledge of man. With the birth of clinical medicine and morbid pathology, surgeons gained access to the insides and once invisible portions of man. With this newfound, internal gaze a discourse emerged that enabled medical professionals to '*see* and to *say*' 'what had previously been beyond and below their domain' (Foucault, 1973, xiii). Over the course of the century, subjective patient narratives were reduced and gradually replaced by analytics within clinicians' reports. Thus began the tradition of the objective medical gaze, resulting in treatments, care practices and consultations that focus heavily on the management of internal factors (such as blood sugar levels), measured through strict numerical indicators. This chapter explores the performance of narrative within the DOC to examine the impact of the clinical gaze for PWD.

Through the clinical gaze, the body of a PWD becomes an object of study, explained and measured through a medical discourse that values an individual's management and control of internal factors. As Frank states, 'Every day society sends us messages that the body can and ought to be controlled. [...] Control is good manners as well as a moral duty; to lose control is to fail socially and morally' (Frank, 1991, 58). PWD negotiate narratives of control and failure when engaging with medical discourses born out of the clinical gaze. Through an examination of performative practices within the DOC, we suggest that PWD are able to perform alternative narratives that provide greater authorial agency for the teller.

As authors of this chapter, we are not criticizing medical professionals for the adoption and implementation of a set of discourses that reduces the body of a patient to an object. Rather, we take inspiration from Frank's assertion that 'the body I experience cannot be reduced to the body someone else measures' (Frank, 1991, 12) to argue that the DOC provides places and platforms where the experience of living with diabetes is performed and alternative narrative practices are adopted. We argue that these narratives provide PWD greater flexibility in how they make sense of their experience of living with diabetes; in turn providing them with greater subjecthood over their bodies and their chronic illness. The multifarious ways in which the DOC presents and represents the bodies and experiences of PWD means that bodies are not merely described: experiences are performed and new discourses emerge.

Undoubtedly, within the DOC, the most common form of engagement and representation of PWD is through patient narratives. Narratives about living with diabetes are narratives of illness, a growing area of study within the medical humanities (see Waddington and Willis, 2013). However, it is not without its critics, who point to the pitfalls of adopting a methodology that is limited and 'unnecessarily restricts what illness narrative might be allowed to mean, and even what it might look like' (Waddington and Willis, 2013, iv). Adopting a performance studies approach enables a deep reading of the illness narratives presented via the DOC.

DOC illness narratives are often non-linear. As our case studies will show, they do not follow traditional story-telling forms based on a linear and progressive structure. They are fragmented, in-situ and ever-evolving documents of experience. They take various forms, ranging from 140 character tweets to lengthy prose; single still images and artwork to vlogs (video blogs) and more traditional performance pieces (dramas and films). The DOC does not simply present stories about how an individual is diagnosed with diabetes, seeks treatment, gains control of the disease, and lives a happy and enriching life thereafter. Rather, the DOC provides a space where individuals are able to present and perform their experiences and worlds, chronicling the ever-fluctuating relationship one has with a chronic illness.

The types of illness narratives performed by PWD via the DOC are different to those that are performed by the clinician during the medical consultation. Similarly, they differ from the public and popular narratives about diabetes, primarily because the patient is able to assert agency over the narration of their experiences, something which is rarely permitted in other contexts. Hazel Morrison references British-American neurologist Oliver Sacks to describe two potential ways of describing the clinical experience: the 'purely nomothetic, "medical" or "classical" [...] objective description' of the illness; and an 'idiographic [...] "existential", "personal empathic entering into patient's experiences and worlds"' (Sacks in Morrison, 2013,18). The DOC mitigates this dichotomy by drawing together and performing both types of description.

Whether the description is the purely medical, numeric measuring of illness, or the more empathic auto-pathological accounts of experiences and worlds, both are stories of illness. One of the ways in which they are distinguished from one another is the extent to which the patient experiences authorial agency over their illness narrative. This is important, as medical humanities scholar Angela Woods argues, because the 'messy and complex subjective experience of illness as something distinct from the biological functioning of disease' requires greater recognition and understanding (Woods, 2013, 38).

Further, recent studies on the UK's 'Expert Patient' programme, aimed at empowering people with the knowledge and skills to effectively manage their chronic conditions, indicate a tension between informed, empowered patients and their healthcare providers (Snow et al., 2013). Combining experiential subjective knowledge with objective bio-medical knowledge, these programmes encourage PWD to emerge as 'empowered...expert patient[s], no longer dependent on doctors for decisions, but able to talk about their treatment requirements with healthcare professionals as an equal' (Snow et al., 2013, 4). The study points to the importance of respecting the expertise gained by patients through this programme and their lived experience. The potential benefits of individual empowerment and 'shared expertise' can 'change people's lives for the better in a way that is perhaps not fully captured by standard clinical and quality of life outcome assessments' (2013, 6). In a sense, the DOC exemplifies another form of patient education, brought out through the shared narratives of lived, experiential, subjective expertise.

Patient narratives are 'neither irrational nor passive but instead [are] actively and subjectively valuable stories of illness that give both meaning and context to the conditions of illness from the patient's perspective' (Willis et al., 2013, 55). The DOC does not necessarily present and perform illness narratives that contest the hegemony of the clinical gaze and associated discourses. Instead, they wrestle with the languages and practices of the clinical gaze and make use of idiosyncratic performance practices to make better sense of their lives as disciplined bodies. We have chosen to provide a detailed, qualitative examination of the content presented and performed by one of the DOCs most avid contributors, Kerri Sparling.

Case study: Kerri Sparling

Kerri Sparling identifies as a writer, speaker and diabetes advocate. Sparling has run the blog *Six Until Me* since May 2005, after growing tired of 'Googling "diabetes" and coming up with little more than a list of complications and frightening stories' (Sparling). When Sparling started blogging, she was one of 'four or five diabetes bloggers' but now, as one of the most prominent voices within the DOC, Sparling's blog is one of many that demonstrate that PWD are not alone in living with their disease (Sparling). Sparling's blog is a mixture of written narratives, images and vlog posts and the themes of connection, acceptance, control, management and an ever fluctuating and evolving relationship with type 1 diabetes stand out as core components.

Sparling makes use of her blog to present and perform her illness narrative. In doing so, she performs the role of expert patient, engaging with medical discourse and the clinical gaze. As such, Sparling's blog grapples with issues of the obedient body and the associated feelings of failure, as well as an uneasy, yet necessary, relationship with being a 'compliant' patient. Through a close reading of the blog, we argue that participation in the DOC has enabled Sparling to transition from what Frank refers to as a position of 'narrative wreckage' to that of an individual with a 'self-story' (Frank, 1995, 55). We focus on five vlog posts that have been produced by, or feature, Sparling, to demonstrate how valuable and important the DOC is in providing PWD the opportunity to create self-stories. Simultaneously, we argue that the type of self-stories performed by Sparling never fully escape the medical discourse, the clinical gaze or the problematic relationship with understanding the body of someone with a chronic disease as a thing to be measured, managed and controlled.

In alignment with narrative theorists, we argue that human beings are storytellers. We live our lives through the stories we perform and the performance of stories informs the type of lives we live. Whenever we perform a story, we do so with a real or imagined audience in mind. Our bodies are essential to our stories. We tell stories about and through our bodies, no more so than when performing illness narratives. Illness narratives have the potential to alter our sense of self as they derail or wreck our narrative trajectories.

For Frank, narrative wreckage occurs when a storyteller loses a sense of temporality, asserting that the 'expectation of any narrative, held alike by listeners and storytellers, is for a past that leads into a present that sets in place a foreseeable future. The illness story is wrecked because its present is not what that past was supposed to lead up to, and the future is scarcely thinkable' (Frank, 1995, 55). Sparling dedicates a section of her blog to sharing the diagnosis stories of her readers and fellow DOC participants. For example, Simon narrates his life, at the point of diagnosis, as feeling like he had built his dream home only for a highway to be built through the middle of it, 'knocking the place down' (Simon in Sparling, 20 May 2007). For Les it is one of confusion, 'What? I don't understand.

What does it mean? That doesn't make any sense. I am literally confused at this point because what he [physician] has said makes no sense' (Les in Sparling, 8 June 2007). For Les and Simon, the memory of diagnosis is presented as a narrative wreck.

In describing why she decided to start blogging about her experiences of living with diabetes, Sparling describes a feeling of isolation and a desire to know if she was the only diabetic 'out there who felt alone' (Sparling). Whilst we are not suggesting that Sparling's blog posts mark the beginning of the DOC, the lack of voices from PWD resulted in a dearth of information about the lived experience of diabetes and a void that was filled with the medical list of complications related to diabetes and horror stories about living with said complications.

In trying to gain understanding about their chronic illness, Sparling, Simon and Les, describe their experiences as bewildering and chaotic. Frank identifies the chaos narrative as a story that 'cannot literally be told but can only be lived' (Frank, 1995, 98). We argue that the experience of living a chaos narrative occurs at numerous points throughout a person's life with diabetes. Most notably, we suggest three main areas where the chaos narrative is experienced: (1) initial diagnosis, (2) the development of diabetes-related complications and (3) the day-to-day fluctuation and turbulence of one's relationship towards the management and control of blood sugar levels. In part, a chaos narrative is propagated by the structure of medical discourse pertaining to diabetes and extenuated through the objectification of the patient and the submission of their voice due to the clinical gaze.

We argue that the voice of the patient is brought in to submission by the way the medical discourse and the clinical gaze work together as a performative structure. The clinician, as expert, adopts a position of authority and power during a consultation. Writing from our lived experience of type 1 diabetes (Pettit) and as the partner of a PWD (Lennox), the authority of the clinician, combined with consultations focused on the observation of internal measurements (blood sugar levels, HBA1C), results in the submission of the patient's voice. The totalizing relationship of the clinical gaze is dominant because the performative structure of the clinical consultation controls and curtails the types of narratives patients can perform. Consultations focus on the current levels of control the PWD has over the management of their illness (determined by blood test results) and the measures they can take to exert greater control. On account of the domineering performative structure of the clinical gaze, the clinical consultation provides little room for the PWD to present narratives that are not focused on control.

However, we do not believe that expert patients provide a counter-narrative to that provided by medical professionals. Through the examples found on Sparling's blog, we demonstrate that PWD are unable to escape the medical discourse, the expertise of their endocrinologists and the clinical gaze. Instead, they engage with performative practices to make sense of their own lived experiences and to add more narrative layers to diabetes discourse.

Authorial agency

Through a close analysis of five videos from Sparling's blog, it is clear that different types of videos solicit different types of illness narrative performances. Whilst all of the selected videos are aimed at PWD, two are shot by and for a manufacturer of diabetes medical equipment. These two videos are of interest not because of their high production value, or because they are commercials, but because they solicit from Sparling a performance of her illness narrative that is markedly different from those of her other videos. The other three videos are vlogs. They have low production value, shot by Sparling in her home. As the two commercial videos are shot for a pharmaceutical company as adverts, they understandably focus more heavily on the numerical indicators associated with the control and management of type 1 diabetes:

> [*Mid-shot of Kerri, in jeans and T-shirt, speaking over an upbeat instrumental bed.*] Hi. I'm Kerri. I've been pumping for eight years, and here's why I love OneTouch Ping. I'm for escaping [*Video cuts to close-up of hands pushing pins into a pin cushion. Over the cushion the text ESCAPING appears.*] one thousand, four hundred and sixty insulin shots. Before I started pumping I was up to nine insulin injections a day. [...]That's actually three thousand, two hundred and eighty five shots a year. I would take them in my arm, my thigh, my stomach, my hips, my butt. It makes you feel like, when you

take a sip of water it is going to come out of all the different holes in your body. The main reason I decided to start pumping was because I knew I wanted to have a baby, and that was the best way for me to gain better control of my diabetes. When I started on the pump, that helped alleviate those lows and my A1C dropped without those hypos.

My endocrinologist knew how hard I was working to lower my A1C, so when we saw the numbers dropping after going on the pump we were both relieved. (Sparling, 2012b)

This narrative performance has a limited focus on the personal experiences and reflections of living with diabetes. Understandably, the narrative performance focuses on the medical benefits derived from the use of the advertised device. Similarly, a second video for the same company features Sparling stressing how important it is to be provided with regular reminders about patterns in her blood sugar levels, 'The easier it is for me to know how I am doing with my numbers, the more confidence I can have throughout the day' (Sparling and Edelman, 2013). We include the excerpts of the commercial videos, not as a critique of Sparling's endorsement of these products, but as an example of how elements of the medical discourse are performed by medical professionals, pharmaceutical companies and patients when they engage with them.

We compare the performance in these videos to that in Sparling's blogs. From a post in September 2011 titled *You Are More Than Diabetes*, Sparling responds to the question, 'What do you wish someone had told you about type 1 diabetes?' In contrast to the professionally produced commercial, this video is clearly self-filmed by Sparling. Throughout the vlog, Sparling speaks with incredible pace, which at times resembles performance poetry. There are numerous cuts and edits to the footage, indicating that the narrative Sparling performs has been refashioned, reformed and carefully considered:

I think one of the things I wish I knew when I was diagnosed – and one of the things I wished I remembered every single day is that these numbers don't define me. There is more to me than just the trail of test strips I leave everywhere. And there is more to me than just the A1C result posted in my logbook. And there is more than just the beeping, and the technology and the focus, focus, focus on what my body doesn't do right. I need to remember that I'm still me underneath all this diabetes stuff. And I'm still me even when my blood sugar is 300. And I'm still me when it's 30. I'm still me. [...]

None of it defines you! None of it is who you are. That these numbers are just measures of my blood sugar, not measures of who I am as a person. (Sparling, 2011)

Numbers still play an important part of Sparling's narrative performance, however, a desire to remember to establish a sense of self outside of the numerical indicators is of greater significance. As the tag line to the blog states, diabetes does not define Sparling, but it does explain her. Within this narrative performance, Sparling seeks to remind herself and her audience that the numbers measure the condition, not the person. Sparling's identity is formed not only in the instances when measurements are being taken, but also in those moments between. Further, the numbers and thus the management of the illness, whilst important, are not to be understood as a measure of the person living with diabetes:

[*Medium close-up of Kerri, wearing a blue top, sat in front of an eggshell background*] I don't know what it is like to live with other diseases, but I do know what it is like to live with type 1 diabetes. And diabetes is a disease that comes with a lot of guilt. [*Kerri's delivery is slower when making the statements regarding numbers and medical complications, but speeds up when posing the questions.*] 'Oh you're 216? Well what did you, what did you eat to make you get that high?' Or, 'Oh! You have diabetic retinopathy in your eye? Well what did you do to get that?' [...] Complications are a result of diabetes, not me! And I [*text appears on the centre, lower third, of screen: 'I barely know what "absolve" means.'*] don't say that to absolve myself of any responsibility. Understanding that diabetes complications are caused by diabetes doesn't enable me. It empowers me. [...] Diabetes is a disease that is more than just the average on your meter or your last A1C result. Understanding those numbers empowers us. But feeling guilty about them and feeling so ashamed of certain results that you don't even react to them. That's not empowerment. That's ... that's awful. Those numbers are important, but the psychosocial aspects of life with diabetes are just as critical. (Sparling, 2012a)

The management of diabetes brings with it a sense of guilt for Sparling. The medical discourse does not adequately account for the psychosocial aspects of life with diabetes. The discourse of control is born out of the medical narratives and the clinical gaze, where social norms suggest that one should manage to assert control over one's own body. Within this context, complications preventing the patient exerting acceptable levels of control mean that the patient has failed to be a 'good' diabetic:

> Complications might come, they might not. But if you get them it doesn't mean that you screwed everything up. It doesn't mean that it is your fault, that you are a bad person. I feel like when people are diagnosed with complications all of a sudden they feel like they have to hide somewhere and you know, they are not allowed to talk about it …. if you are diagnosed with something difficult or a complication or something that people are thinking you're suppose to be able to avoid, you are suppose to keep your voice quiet. You're supposed to keep your story to yourself. (Sparling, 2014)

By engaging with the medical discourse and her personal illness narrative, Sparling performs a self-story about her lived experience of chronic illness. Her narrative differs slightly, dependent upon whether the video is self-filmed or shot in collaboration with medical experts. There is a subtle subversion of the gaze when Kerri authors her vlogs, over those videos where the message, script and material is shot and edited by someone else. However, at no point does Sparling's narrative reject the expertise of her medical team and the problematics inherent to adopting their narrative practices and a discourse that objectifies the patient's body through the clinical gaze.

Conclusion

> The body is not to be managed, even by myself. My body is a means and medium of my life; I live not only in my body but also through it. No one should be asked to detach his mind from his body and then talk about this body as a thing, out there. (Frank, 1991, 10)

Within the medical narratives about diabetes is a degree of universality, wherein normative numeric ranges (for things such as A1C counts and glucose levels) govern what constitutes a 'good' diabetic patient. Through the clinical narratives offered by physicians and medical professionals, PWD are constantly reminded to aim for a specific and limited set of numeric indicators. These numbers can be difficult to achieve and do not necessarily best reflect the complexities and diversities of the lives of PWD. As a result, PWD can routinely feel a sense of failure, guilt and shame when engaging with medical professionals.

The DOC offers a site where PWD are able to engage with the universal precept of diabetes management. Through the narrative accounts of their lived experience with diabetes, contributors to the DOC are able to challenge, refuse and contest the universal, by offering the personal and the individual as counter narratives. The lived experience of PWD is performed, consumed and adopted by the DOC. An expertise different to that offered by medical professions lies at the heart of the DOC. It is central to the success of the community and is the site where the true value of the DOC can really be measured. Failure to witness, accept and respond to the diversity of performed expertise by PWD is a violent rejection of subjecthood. The value of the DOC can best be measured when diverse perspectives and voices are engaged in discourse about living with, treating and managing responses to the day to day experiences of a chronic illness.

When performing an illness narrative about living with diabetes, patients are likely to perform different types of stories to different audiences. The illness narrative that one tells to the clinician is likely to differ in content and structure to that told to a close friend, relative or fellow members of the DOC. The difference in the content and structure outlined in the examples above demonstrate how different audiences solicit different narrative performances. However, what the case study demonstrates is that when telling an illness narrative about diabetes it is impossible to escape the medical discourse. Medical terminology and language structures are embedded within the stories. As such, the clinical gaze, wherein the patient's body is objectified through the expertise of the physician's analysis, remains a dominant feature of diabetes illness narratives in the DOC. The narratives performed by the DOC are unable to reject the expertise of the medical professions, nor do they aspire to do so.

That said, the DOC provides a space where individuals can engage with illness narratives and the medical discourse in a way that allows PWD to reclaim authorial agency over their own stories and lived experience of diabetes. The narratives that PWD perform through the DOC are not counter narratives to those provided by medical professionals. Instead, they make personal and accessible experiences of living with diabetes for fellow members of the online community. The DOC provides platforms and spaces where the narrative wreckage associated with initial diagnosis, the development of diabetes-related complications, or the day-to-day fluctuation and turbulence of one's relationship towards the management and control of blood sugar levels, can be mitigated through narration. Thus, the DOC provides individuals with the opportunity to develop beyond a chaos narrative to a self-story with greater flexibility in terms of the types of lives it enables one to perform.

8

Cough, Bitch, Cough: Reflections on Sickness and the Coughing Body in Performance

Martin O'Brien

The train was at the platform when I dashed down the stairs and jumped into the back carriage just before the doors closed. I was late for an interview about my work – it was a few days after my 2012 performance *Regimes of Hardship #1*. I was out of breath when I reached an empty seat. I sat down and there was a man in front of me wearing a suit. I was breathing heavily and started to cough. I suffer from the life-shortening chronic illness cystic fibrosis (CF), a disease in which the body over-produces bodily fluids, particularly mucus. So coughing is a major part of my daily existence. When I cough from exercise it doesn't tend to be a small polite cough, rather one of those lung-racking, bone-shaking coughs. You can almost hear phlegm. It is the sound of cystic fibrosis. It is the sound of disease. After a few minutes, the man in front stood up, sighed loudly so that I could hear him, and moved to another seat as far away from me as he could get.

We might think of his action as understandable: to move yourself away from the perceived threat of contamination. It seems to be learnt culturally that avoiding contact with diseased people is necessary to remain healthy. Indeed, there are many historical contexts in which infected people were forced into restricted situations in order to prevent contagion.[1] The cough itself is a sign of illness; it is the sound sick people make. But it is also a way in which illness passes from one person to another. It is a warning

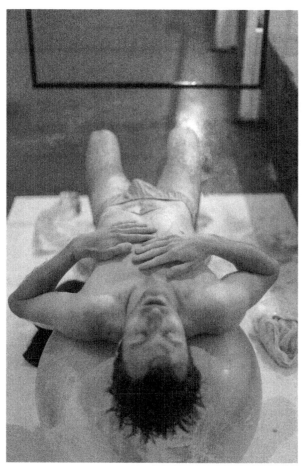

FIGURE 8.1 *Martin O'Brien*, Regimes of Hardship #1 *(2012). Photo by Marco Berardi.*

sign, the way in which one body tells another 'I'm sick' and the other responds by avoiding contiguity or escaping the possibly noxious environment causing the cough. With CF the cough is something that occurs daily. However, while it does function as a signal of the disease there is no possibility of infection. Its function, philosophically, is different. However, the cough seems to demand the reaction of separation. A human does not want to be near the cough of another.

Simon Bayly suggests that 'the cough plagues the theatre as an obstacle to performance, evident in the clearing of the airway prior to the commencement of song and its pathological corollary in the extended coughing fits of audiences between acts or movements' (Bayly, 2011, 168). The cough marks a rupture; it is uncontrollable. But what is at stake when the cough *is* the performance, rather than an introduction to, or interruption of, it? Or when the cough is something striven for within performance? My entire oeuvre of work tends to be punctuated by fits of coughing. Performances such as *Mucus Factory* (2011–2014), *Regimes of Hardship* (2012), *Breathe For Me* (2012–2015) and *Last(ing)* (2013) have all included actions designed to induce coughing. I will first briefly define what a cough is in practical terms before considering my philosophical concerns around the cough and performance.

Philosophy of the cough

In his book *Paralanguage*, linguist Fernando Poyatos borrows from his research into medical physiology to describe the cough as a:

> violent reflex air release from the lungs triggered, for instance, by irritation by foreign matter of the larger air-passages (i.e. bronchi, trachea and vocal folds), or by inflammation of the lining mucous membrane of the bronchi and trachea. During a cough the epiglottis, as well as the glottis in the vocal folds...close tightly after air is inspired, then the abdominal, intercoastal and other muscles contract forcefully, immediately after which the air pushes the glottis and epiglottis open explosively. Some books say 'a deep breath is taken'...yet we know that many

times the explosive, spasmodic reflex is triggered instantly and uncontrollably before we can attempt to draw in any air at all, a cough that, so to speak, surprises even the cougher. (Poyatos, 1993, 347)

Poyatos outlines that within physiology the cough is always a surprise. What impact does this have upon our understanding of the cough and how it functions within performance? Bayly points to the cough as something which has been ignored by philosophy, suggesting that the 'cough is the "creature voiced", but also what molests the vocal organs, barely fit for thought, let alone philosophy. Philosophy has sought to erase the cough, to eradicate its interruptive force' (Bayly, 2011, 166–7). He continues by highlighting 'Aristotle's rejection of the cough as merely the impact of the breath' and Husserl's 'consignment of all paralinguistics or kinesis expression to the category of the meaningless' as examples of 'philosophy's repulsion for the organic process of vocalization' (2011, 167). Little thought has been given to the cough, which, like its sister, the sneeze, is seen as both a symbol and effect of illness. One might think of the popular rhyming slogan taken from the 1945 public health poster and film: *coughs and sneezes spread diseases* used to teach people to cover their mouth when they do either (Massingham).

In his study of the voice, David Appelbaum suggests that a 'cough is the detonation of voice' (Appelbaum, 1990, 2). If the cough is the detonation of voice, though, it is equally the forceful establishment of a different voice, one which does not adhere to language – the voice of illness. The cough interrupts, it is something that cannot be contained and demands its right to be heard. It functions as a disordering of the voice and of the breath. Appelbaum continues thinking about the nature of the cough:

It is duller than the pierce of a cry which goes to the heart. On the terminal ward, one hears the cries first. But the coughs penetrate more deeply, into the compact soma of the body. There they contact an organic memory which reminds us of death and life as facts unembellished by feelings. If the world were cured of the common cough, we would be less prepared for our earthly passage. (Appelbaum, 1990, 2)

The cough seems to initiate our deepest bodily identification. It is as if the cough speaks directly to the flesh of others, like a warning siren, triggering bodily memories of coughing in times of illness. If the coughing fit has the potential to spark fear of infection within others it equally holds within it the possibility of empathy. These possibilities seem to emerge from the way in which the common rhetoric surrounding the cough has been framed, which means that the mere sound of it signals danger. There is a reluctance to be near the cougher. I would propose, developing from Appelbaum, that a fear of illness drives this. If the cough 'reminds us of death and life' (Appelbaum, 1990, 2) then it is something to be avoided, as it reminds us of the potential of death within life. It becomes a threat to our health and ultimately our existence.

Performance and the coughing body

If the cough is seen as a threat because of its potential for the spread of sickness, how might I understand my coughing body in performance? Far from being something that plagues performance, as Bayly suggests, the cough is something intrinsic to the nature of my work. What does the act of coughing in front of an audience do, particularly when spectators are aware that the coughing body is a chronically sick one? The cough is both something caused by endurance, the endurance of illness and of the physically demanding activity being performed, and something to be endured itself. As such, it holds a critical position within the performance of sickness. As someone with CF, I cough when I exercise but throughout the duration of the performance the cough itself becomes an act of endurance: the endless expelling of air, the drying up of the throat, the taste of mucus, the loss of an articulate voice. Relentless coughing removes the possibility of speech; instead the cough establishes itself as the voice of illness. The cough in these performances, then, is both a symptom, of sickness and endurance, and, at the same time, a cause.

My coughing body demonstrates the potential to infect, even if it is not actually possible. This has implications for understanding spectatorship within my performances specifically, but also more generally for the work of artists with illness who ask viewers to share the same space with them. Attitudes towards the coughing body are symptomatic of societal attitudes towards the sick body and thus by focusing closely upon this and the fear it induces I will be able to examine what it means to view the sick body in performance. The sick body is identified as posing risk and the cough is a way of warning of this risk. The coughing body, then, is always presumed to be a body capable of spreading disease. Moreover, the idea of contagion provides a useful metaphor for considering the relationship between the sick body in performance and the spectators. I suggest that these works dis-ease the onlookers through a form of contact (Hannah, 2007, 135). My own coughing body in performance plays upon a deep-rooted fear of contagion. I signal myself as sick in performances, during which my body spills out in the form of the cough and the mucus produced by it. The excessive amount of this bodily fluid marks me out as sick. In these moments, my sickness is revealed. In life I am able to 'pass' as healthy. I don't look or act sick.

A description of my own personal experience of coughing within the performance offers a reflection upon the visibility of sickness in performance. After beating my chest with my hands there is an eruption: the sound of the cough penetrates the bodies in the space with me and the phlegm gushes from inside my body; from the deepest depths of my lungs comes a thick bright green/yellow substance that is both part of me and killing me. My body convulses, my face turns red as I struggle to control the cough, or to prevent the mucus from flying out of my mouth. I catch it in my hands: I feel its warm wet viscous texture and taste what can only be described as 'mucusy'. I hold cystic fibrosis in my hands. My fluids point towards my body as being sick.

I think about the man on the train and his dis-ease with my sick body, his movement away could be read as 'a shrinking from contamination' (Nussbaum, 2004, 74). In this instance, we may understand dis-ease in relation to disgust:

> The disgusted person turns away from the offending sight or smell, driven by a desire to avoid all contact and to minimise cognisance of that which is perceived as disgusting. Disgust is an aversion not just to the physical touch of an entity, but its essence. Objects of disgust are viewed as contagious, transferring

their unwanted properties to things which they are associated
and affecting people through sights or smells and, less often,
sounds. (Cushing and Markwell, 2010, 168)

The cough is, fundamentally, a sound. Cushing and Markwell
suggest here that the contagion associated with disgusting objects
are considered as contagious more often not only through sight
and smell but also sound. The sound of coughing seems to dis-ease
through the way it is able to speak directly to the flesh of other
humans. The sound of another human coughing causes physical
responses of our own. The man on the train was so irritated or
concerned by the sound of my cough behind him that he had to
move.

I propose that, in performance, the sick body causes disgust
and it is this feeling that causes conservative reactionary responses
to difficult practices emerging from a refusal or inability to
comprehend the value of a work. As the mucus-covered coughing
body, I am marked as deviant Other. Not only sick because of illness
but the way in which I manage this sickness is sick. It is difficult to
valorize my use of my body in this way within a society governed
by an ideology of health and in which bodily fluids are seen as
contaminants to be avoided, certainly not presented within an
aesthetic framework:

The fundamental schema of disgust is the experience of a nearness
that is not wanted. An intrusive presence, a smell or taste is
spontaneously assessed as contamination and forcibly distanced.
The theory of disgust, to that extent, is a counterpart – although
not a symmetrical one – of the theory of love, desire and
appetite as forms of intercourse with a nearness that is wanted.
(Menninghaus, 2003, 1)

My sick coughing body is disgusting because it poses the threat
of contamination. The leaky sick body, unable to control the
spillage of its bodily fluids, in an art context repels but also presents
itself as something to be looked at. For Ngai, disgust serves as an
aesthetic emotion and trapped within the schema of disgust is the
paradox that 'what makes the object abhorrent is precisely its
outrageous claim for desirability. The disgusting seems to say, "You

want me", imposing itself on the subject as something to be mingled with and perhaps even enjoyed' (Ngai, 2005, 335). The spectators, by remaining in the space, allow themselves to be contaminated. They invite the dis-ease of witnessing the sick, enduring body. It is this form of contact which prevents the viewer reading a work as representational and instead they become hyper-aware of their own body and its relationship to that of the artist. Just being with the deviant sick body pollutes the body of the viewer. As an embodied being, a dis-eased spectator is reminded of the materiality of their own body through an engagement with the flesh, blood, mucus of another. Disgust may function as a defence mechanism against the dis-ease caused by this contagion but, as Ngai noted, one is both repelled and drawn to the object of disgust.

A spectator makes the choice to remain in the room watching the sick body. To view this work is to acknowledge the need to be dis-eased by the Other. Unlike the man on the train who moved away from me, the spectators of my work choose contact. They are drawn to the fragility of another human being but repelled by its sickness, by the actual material of a body slowly dying. Christian Moraru suggests that 'viruses communicate themselves, the same information or, better still, the same as information' (Moraru, 2012, 129). In the same way, the contagion of sick performance then communicates sickness. It communicates that the body you are watching is sick and that you, as a viewer and embodied being, are also sick or soon will be. It acts as a reminder that sickness is unavoidable, no matter what defence mechanisms are in place, and that this existence is contingent upon the maintenance of our physical body. The dis-ease of understanding this through contact with this art of sickness is compelling and necessary but difficult and sometimes, even, unbearable.

PART THREE

Performing Body Parts

9

The Pain of 'Specimenhood'

Gianna Bouchard

Western medical science has a long history of displaying bodies for the purposes of examination, diagnosis, treatment, research and education. Looking at the body in order to understand it and to identify its ailments and pathologies, to compare healthy parts with diseased ones, and comprehend its intricate workings, has always been a part of medical practice. But the early medical gaze soon faltered on the superficial and relatively uninformative exposure of the outside of the body and its various appearances, expulsions and excretions. So medical ocular desire turned inwards, to the layers beneath the skin, the organs and anatomy of the body, and to what the interior might reveal about the subject and their biological functioning. Physicians turned their attention, whenever possible, to seeing below the skin and within the body, leading to the development of the practice of anatomical dissection from the fourteenth century onwards.[1]

At the centre of dissective practice, as Jonathan Sawday notes, is a 'stress on direct, visual, sensory experience that involves "the cultivation of autopsia" – literally, seeing for oneself' (1995, 35). During the early modern period this became a public and spectacular moment of display of the body, where intimate looking at the body was enabled through the use of purpose-built anatomy theatres. Medical men and the public sought to understand human physiology through these demonstrations and to witness, as they perceived it at the time, God's divine creation, by and through anatomical demonstration. At the centre of the physical and intellectual space of the anatomy theatre was the corpse, the human specimen, raised into sight on a table or platform, and dissected according to a strict order, and within a tight temporal framework. Death is not static or fixed in these moments, but is a fluid and mutable condition that alters the body through decay and decomposition, so the dissectors had to work efficiently and effectively to beat the onset of putrefaction, which can quickly render the body useless for these anatomical demonstrations.

Alongside the need to divide the body and examine its interior, there arose an understandable desire to preserve it, so that 'autopsia', exposure and interrogation could be extended beyond the brief window of opportunity immediately after death. Inevitably, anatomists have long experimented with different methods of preserving disaggregated body parts for further study and research. The impetus, as medical historian Sam Alberti puts it, to 'freeze time', to render the 'indistinct visible, the ephemeral durable' and the need to provide a 'permanent reference point' about bodies and their pathologies is borne out in the extensive collections of specimens held and maintained by medical museums across the country (2011, 6).

The specimen, according to the *Oxford English Dictionary*, can be 'a part or portion of something that can serve as an example of the thing in question, for the purpose of investigation or scientific study'. It can also be a single thing, selected or regarded as typical of its class, a part of something that is taken as representative of the whole. From the literal fragmented part, the specimen also stands as an example in a philosophical and intellectual sense. Derived from the Latin word '*specere*', meaning 'to look' or 'to look at', the specimen depends on some kind of radical separation from the original whole, in order for it to be more fully observed, analysed and considered as an exemplar and a demonstration or test case. It can be both an example, in and of itself, and representative of a particular type or class of something. In this chapter, the specimen will be considered as both a physical entity, in relation to the medical practice of excising and preserving body parts and pathologies, and as a conceptual tool, in order to briefly consider a growing context of practices that create specimens in the contemporary moment. More specifically, the idea of the specimen will be explored in relation to performance through Clod Ensemble's 2010 *Under Glass*.

The specimens examined here are literal, in the performance, but they also enable, or are embedded in, a conceptual methodology of 'specimenhood'. This notion comes from Gladstone and Berlo's essay on museums and the ethical issues that arise from displaying bodies within those contexts (2011). They are particularly interested in the relatively recent phenomenon of the artist's body being staged in museums (such as that of Marina Abramovic) and believe the concept of specimenhood to be an 'essential consideration in conceptualising an ethics of the body on display' (Gladstone and Berlo, 2011, 354). By adopting this analytical approach, I hope to analyse *Under Glass* in order to reflect back on wider issues of constructions of specimens in culture, on issues of spectatorship and the ethics of display. Finally, I will consider the potential of performance to make us think differently about our encounters with specimens.

Clod Ensemble, founded and directed by Suzy Willson and Paul Clark, is a London-based company that produces theatre and performance work that focuses on exploring relations between music and movement. Part of their work has explicit connections to performance and medicine, particularly in their project *Performing Medicine*. This brings medical personnel, academics and wider publics into dialogue with each other through performance workshops, talks and direct engagements with the medical curriculum and the education of doctors at various teaching hospitals in London.[2] Works such as *Under Glass* and *An Anatomie in Four Quarters* deliberately bring these two strands of theatre and medicine together.

Under Glass was made up of eight individual dance and movement-based performances that were brought together in 2010 for a national tour and, as part of the tour, was shown at the Village Underground in Shoreditch, London. Each performance was contained within a different shaped specimen jar, one of which was specifically named as a 'test tube' and another that appears to be a circular Petri dish. There was also a 'jam jar', and various square containers of different heights, widths and depths. Each contained a solo performer throughout the piece, with the exception of the 'twins', who shared the circular container.[3] The programme notes for the work directly reference the idea that the piece was 'at once museum exhibit, gallery and medical laboratory' and so implying that these performers, in their transparent containers, were, in some way, staged as specimens (Willson and Clark, 2010).

Under Glass invited its audience into the darkened warehouse in Shoreditch, and there isolated performers in their various jars and containers, spread throughout the space and presented on different levels, confronted us. The initial moments of the work slowly revealed several of the performers, bringing the lights up gradually on their confinements and producing shadowy glimpses of bodies, faces and parts. As an audience member, I steadily realized that there were multiple specimens and the space emerged as reminiscent of a medical museum or an exhibition of captured individuals. The lighting gradually enabled a more focused gaze at the specimens and their jars became apparent too, as we caught sight of reflections and edges that began to be definable as transparent vessels. Sitting and standing in the darkness, the specimens were drawn attention to, highlighted and emphasized through the lighting, so that they emerged from and disappeared back into the darkness. In their slow revelation, the 'lo and behold' of science and performance mingled, presenting bodies and performers to be looked at, to be seen, deciphered and offered to contemplation.

Evoking medico-science's concerns with identifying, examining, preserving and collecting specimens as material for demonstration, revelation, examination and research, the work played across the idea of the specimen as both sample and exemplar. Seemingly separated from their original contexts and caught in their containers, the performers were offered as specimens, valued for their potential to provoke new insights, whilst also being a bio-archive and record of certain human conditions; conditions of human existence, rather than disease, such as the worker trapped in his too-small office, surrounded by post-it notes, and struggling to contain his boredom and sense of growing frustration at the monotony of it all. They were transformed biological artefacts and enduring – like the medical specimen – into an unknown and ongoing future of containment, testing, display and spectacularization.

In terms of medicine and science, the removal, storage and future use of the specimen is framed by complex social, cultural, epistemological, medical and legal concerns that make them highly charged and multifaceted objects in certain contexts.[4] So, for instance, within public discourse in the UK, little seems to be said about the display of mummified human remains from archaeological sites or collected as part of ethnographic research, when presented within the museum or gallery. The Egyptian mummies in the British

Museum, for example, remain the most popular exhibit in the collections but, on the other hand, we have witnessed significant political, social and ethical furore around more recently revealed and, apparently hitherto, 'secret' specimens kept by medical institutions. Or, indeed, there has been disapproval and outright condemnation of the creation of human specimens that appear to be spectacularized in undignified and inappropriate ways, such as in the touring exhibition of plastinated cadavers and body parts in the *Bodyworlds* show; the anatomical exhibition, created by maverick scientist Gunther von Hagens.

The early twenty-first century has certainly seen increased public anxiety about medical research and practices that appear to create specimens without consent or attention to the ethical dilemmas of extending and manipulating biological materials outside of the original body. For instance, in 1999, the British public's attention was drawn to a growing scandal centred on Alder Hey Children's Hospital, Liverpool, where children's organs were being removed and stored by a senior pathologist, for which there was no parental consent. Such storage creates enduring body specimens for medico-science but, in this instance, the controversy sparked debates about rights over ownership of the body and informed consent. As I have noted elsewhere, 'in an attempt to close some of the legal loopholes, to ensure protection of patient's rights and to improve ethical standards in biomedical practice, UK civil legislation followed the Bristol and Alder Hey organ retention inquiries with the revised Human Tissue Act of 2004' (Bouchard, 2012, 100–101). This law 'sought to clarify the regulation of biological materials removed from dead and living bodies. Based on the principal of consent, it rendered illegal the removal and storage of human tissue and organs without appropriate, informed consent, and it outlawed organ trafficking and DNA theft' (2012, 101).[5]

In more recent times, the constellation of practices that create specimens has, arguably, escaped from the narrow confines of medicine and entered into mainstream culture, often dragging medico-scientific discourses in its wake, ever a prop to the use of the specimen, and a legitimating frame for its display. Often, the medical or scientific is used to frame extraordinary bodies in a way that seems to sanction, authorize and encourage our viewing, which in other contexts might be deemed to be inappropriate or even voyeuristic. Spectatorial desire and encouragement to look at bio-specimens remains (finding its roots in the early modern anatomical theatres and in the Victorian 'freak shows') and has even been heightened in some medical contexts, in popular culture and in performative terms. Gunther von Hagens, the creator of the *Bodyworlds* exhibition of plastinated corpses and body parts, said 'you have to recognize yourself as a specimen' (von Hagens in Gladstone and Berlo, 2011, 353). This could, rather chillingly, refer to a desire, on his part, to see us all as potential donors and participants in his exhibitions. In other words, that we are ripe for plastinating at some point in his anatomizing future and that each of us could reveal something instructive about human anatomy. But, I think, it also draws us to consider the current status of the body and its spectacularization in mainstream culture, where 'everyday', non-normative physiologies and anatomies are being transformed into specimens of 'embarrassing bodies'. Such bodies are in need of correcting, curing and normalizing, once they have been identified as potential specimens and in need of professional, usually medical, help.

For instance, some television shows, such as Channel 4's *Embarrassing Bodies* (2007–ongoing) and *Supersize vs. Superskinny* (2008–ongoing), seem to convert the ordinary person into a medical specimen, and thereby the shows reiterate the notion of these individuals as being both samples and exemplars. In discussing ethnographic objects in the museum, Kirshenblatt-Gimblett describes the method of showing such artefacts as being dependent on 'an art of excision, of detachment' and likens the process of selection to a surgical procedure (1998, 18). It requires a kind of cut that separates the object from the original body or site. This is a violent manoeuvre, an excision and a rending, but it is also about separation and fragmentation. In many ways, we can see a version of this in these medical reality programmes, as the specimen is identified as needing attention and is often removed from or detached from their everyday situations, in order to become the object of study. They are transported to a special location, in laboratories or medicalized spaces, where they are scrutinized, tested and provoked to become healthier and to discipline themselves into improved living practices. Surveillance of their bodies is often highly intrusive, with 360-degree views of their bodies and, sometimes, including scans and X-rays of their inner selves. The living specimen is visually disaggregated in front of our eyes and then, apparently, put back together again or, at least, is put back onto the straight and narrow of self-transformation and 'cure' by the end of each programme. In these instances, we can see that the body, displayed as a specimen, is a powerful tool and support to discourses around normativity; for reinforcing the status and power of science and medicine; and, for encouraging self-surveillance, self-monitoring and disciplinary practices in the wider population.

Clod Ensemble's specimens were, likewise, isolated and vulnerable, separated from each other and from the audience by their various containers, which are a key part of the preservation of medical specimens. The jars limited their freedoms and their movements, whilst also being the means of experimenting with those limits – the performers struggled within the spaces, pushed against the glass, used it to support their weight and reach to their limits. They simultaneously posed, measured and tested themselves within their confines. At times, the specimen-performers seemed to be aware that their bodies and selves were on show and they proceeded to demonstrate themselves, in a manner that recalls pictorial representations from the seventeenth and eighteenth centuries of dissected bodies. These figures were involved in showing the body as the spectacle of the unseen and were active participants in their own revelation, often holding back their skin, like drapes, in order to display their internal organs for the viewer. They were also invariably drawn in action, against striking landscapes, seemingly proud and acquiescent in their own dismemberment. Jonathan Sawday describes this principle as that of 'living anatomy', where dissected subjects were represented as being alive and fully participant in the dissective process (1995, 114). Clod Ensemble's performers sometimes echoed such self-demonstrations, appearing to want to show themselves and aware of their 'to be looked at-ness', pressing flesh to glass and pointing towards the audience. In these moments, the performer-specimens were complicit in their own display, comfortable in themselves and in their own revelation. In other moments, though, a different dynamic was revealed, where the performers seemed acutely uncomfortable in their presentation and hesitant or introverted in their containers. Still others performed as though entirely unaware that they were being looked at, and were caught up in their own struggles with their environments, as though the glass was an opaque barrier and edge to their worlds.

For the audience, watching *Under Glass* meant being involved in this exchange of looks and gazes. In the programme notes, Kélina Gotman describes the experience of watching it as 'uncanny'. The work 'shifts the gaze, makes us squint, wonder, turn our heads this way and that, to gain a new perspective, a new slant, a new angle' (2010). Following the work of Rosemarie Garland-Thomson, the specimen is often staged within a 'scene of staring', where the starer tries to understand the unfamiliar object and thereby master it, which requires the 'arduous visual work of reconciling the curious with the common' (2009, 49). The display of the specimen within science and medicine is often predicated on the incitement of curiosity in the viewer, which then provokes a resultant search for new knowledge and understanding. Curiosity, in these contexts, is considered a noble impulse, which draws the viewer close to the object in an intense visual scrutiny that supposedly orders, categorizes and enables a gradual knowing of the subject.

In writing about curiosity, Barbara Benedict suggests that the objects of museums and cabinets of curiosities, in other words, collections of specimens, 'make readers both curious consumers and consumers of curiosity' (2001, 9). Specimens establish a complex relational dynamic between the 'curious' object and the spectator:

> Like images in a hall of mirrors replicating their reflections, curious spectators inhabit simultaneously the roles of inquirer and object of inquiry, watching themselves watching, and creating ever more curious consumers. This solipsistic aspect makes curiosity vulnerable to the host of moral charges traditionally associated with narcissism (2001, 9).

The specimen inaugurates a constant slippage for the viewer between spectator and performer, between subject and object, which implies a certain spectatorial pleasure in this shifting economy. *Under Glass* engaged in these economies by leading the audience round the space, to encounter the specimens from a variety of perspectives and in a manner that incited a certain kind of curiosity. The slow revelation of the performers in their jars certainly invoked anticipation and inquisitiveness, as we couldn't quite see enough to fully determine what we were being shown, at least at first. Some of the specimens were very close, whilst others were distant and raised up, and some were below us, lying down and morphing into strange shapes, as though under a microscope. The 'look of curiosity' was explored here but in a way that diminished its power over the specimen-performers. As Gotman states, '[w]e watch, without judging' (2010). The audience were aware of others sharing this look, and we could often see others watching and 'watching themselves watching' but the violence of the stare was prohibited. Kuppers describes the visualization techniques involved in medicine and, more particularly, in practices of anatomy as the 'violence of the vision machine of anatomy' (2004, 133). This violence was evoked in the work but simultaneously negated into an empathic and shared encounter.

This looking, that was encouraged by the performance, played between a kind of forbidden staring at bodies that was sanctioned in this space and an intense pleasure in watching the performers. The lights were never increased enough to replicate the glare of the laboratory or the spotlight of the museum or gallery, and nor were they harsh enough to fully render the subjects in exacting detail. The play of light and shadow that framed and located each container negated the analytical power of the medical gaze. There was no thrusting into the spotlight or complete revelation that might have laid these performers bare. They remained partially enigmatic and ephemeral beings, who had not been preserved or held in stasis by the processes of transformation usually deployed on medical specimens. They were living, changing and 'being' in front of us, if only for the forty minutes of the performance: 'The human specimens, doing their working, dancing, sleeping, reconfigured so that what we are looking at are just simply lives' (Gotman, 2010). Subjugation and violence were subverted from the scene in favour of an ethical looking that was tender and gentle.

This ethical engagement was produced, in part, by the scenography and lighting, but also by the performers, their movements, and their individual subjectivities, which were manifest in the work. The medical museum and the pathological specimen suppress the individual 'to the structuring process of the scientific gaze, exposing muscles and flesh, not individuality' (Kuppers, 2004, 137). Medico-science's work with specimens involves a process of rendering the body into what Alberti defines as 'material culture' (2011, 100). In the journey from anatomization and fragmentation to specimen, the individual shifts from subject to object, 'from him or her to *it*' (2011, 95) and contemporary anxieties about medicine and science are often focused on these kinds of dehumanizing elements. The storage of body parts without consent, the use of cell lines for development and financial gain, and the trade in organs, have all raised social anxieties about the potential for the individual to become distanced or separated from their own body, and, in turn, raising questions about property rights and ownership of our bodies. There is a growing concern about what medical ethicist Alistair Campbell describes as the 'potential dehumanization of the self, by treating it as no more than a rational negotiator in a society dominated in all its aspects by market values, including the monetizing of parts of the human body' (2009, 18).

Clod Ensemble's work, however, presented specimens as and of everyday life, recognizable in all their fragility and idiosyncrasies, who were hauntingly familiar in their habits, frustrations and expressions of limitation. Where the medical specimen is fragmented, separated and potentially dehumanized, these specimens were warm, animated and extraordinary. In some ways, this signals the pain of 'specimenhood' and we may begin to realize the implications of singling out people and parts, of categorizing, of labelling, of separating, of isolating, of testing, of analysing and displaying each other. The work encouraged an ethics of care in these moments, by inviting connections and reciprocity across physical, social, philosophical and cultural divides. These bodies were 'empathized with, felt and cared for' (Gotman, 2010).

Interwoven with the movement in the piece is Alice Oswald's poem *The Village*, which was specifically written for the work and is spoken into a telephone by the performer in a test tube, and Paul Clark's original music. The poem speaks of fragments of village life, offering snapshots of events and behaviours in an analogous manner to the construction of the specimen, snippets lifted from their originary context and framed as both example and exemplar. The poem names certain individuals in the fictional village, such as John Strong and Joyce Jones, describing their seemingly clandestine behaviours and revealing snatches of brutal and violent scenes, played out at night and in the dark, glimpsed through windows or down darkened country lanes. Spied on and described on the telephone to an unknown other, these are more familiar specimens of our daily lives, separated out, gossiped about and turned into the victims of rumours. But there is also the repeated refrain of 'good grief you get used to the sound' (Oswald, 2010), creating a sense that we are desensitized to certain moments of brutality and cruelty, which we inflict on each other. This threading through of a text about individual lives and their experiences of pain, and even death and murder, of fractured relationships and loneliness, connects us to the performer-specimens and each other, revivifying our shared humanity.

The specimen relies upon this construction of relations between bodies to become meaningful, including in the medical collection. In the museum, as Alberti points out, the collection is a 'dynamic entity, a set of relations enacted through material' that comprises biological specimens, models, images, texts and other connected objects, such as surgical instruments and other medical paraphernalia (2011, 7). The specimen is made sense of through its relationality to other specimens and means of anatomical representation. Excised and detached, it is given significance through its association with other fragmented parts, divided but then situated within another complex body of parts. This relationality is prevalent in many of the moments of specimenhood I have begun to identify here. The early modern anatomical dissection was dependent on a single material body but underpinned very explicitly by a relation to authoritative textual bodies, spoken over the dissective process and used to highlight the veracity of the anatomy text. The anatomized specimen was also displayed alongside the anatomical drawing, in a didactic and mutually reinforcing system of representations. Arguably, this is also present in the spectacle of televised specimens, where bodies are compared to other bodies, real and idealized, pathologized and normative. Their transgressions are made apparent when they are related to other, more disciplined and apparently more civil bodies. This is, of course, extended to a relation with the body of the viewer, who is drawn into and encouraged to make comparisons between the screened specimen and the body on the sofa. Relations are established, which reflect back and forth between viewer and specimen, that should either apparently encourage the viewer to seek similar medical help or take action, or that offers spectatorial pleasure (and it is surely more of this than the former) realizing that 'one's position on the far side of the stage is assured' (Kuppers, 2003, 35). Pleasure and satisfaction comes from establishing that 'I am not like that', where the relation is constructed through difference, rather than sameness.

It is here that *Under Glass* subverts these systems of representation, as I have been arguing. Instead of believing that we are not the same as the specimens in their various containers, the work draws us to recognize that such differences are constructed, often condemnatory and ethically dubious. The exchange of relations in the performance subtly shift the focus back to the self and the body of the spectator, as the origin of the enduring specimen, as the material that matters, when medicine and science appear to work in the opposite direction. It is performance practice that returns us to the fragile, vulnerable and divisible body that appears to be increasingly manipulated, commodified and exploited by some biotechnologies, which are able to make the body, our bodies and its parts endure into unknown futures.

Novelist Hilary Mantel wrote about medical museums in 2010: 'in old-fashioned museums you can see the unconscious benefactors of mankind, trapped in glass cases: the freaks and monsters of their day ... When we look at them, fascination and repulsion uneasily mixed, we bow our heads to their contribution to knowledge, but it is hard to locate their humanity' (Mantel in *Guardian Review,* May 2010, 7). It seems to me that Clod Ensemble's work draws us back towards an ethics of care and responsibility for those identified as specimens and it reflects on the processes of specimenhood, which seem to be increasingly prevalent in a constellation of practices, some of which I have identified here. Presented with dignity and warmth, these specimens are fleshy, lonely and struggling selves, and the weight of ethical responsibility falls on the spectator. *Guardian* reviewer, Sanjoy Roy, tellingly reveals this weight when he notes: 'At the end, ... when they turn inside their cabinets to look at us, applauding from within our own patch of light, it is as if we are the lonely weirdos, not them' (Roy, 2009).

10

Clod Ensemble, *An Anatomie in Four Quarters* Rehearsal Notes

Suzy Willson

An Anatomie in Four Quarters is a performance piece by Clod Ensemble, first performed at Sadler's Wells theatre in 2011. Here, Artistic Director Suzy Willson shares some rehearsal notes about the piece. This is not intended as a script or record of the performance but as a description of some of the ideas that inform it.

OVERVIEW

An Anatomie in Four Quarters is:
An anatomy of a theatre

An anatomy of the study of anatomy

An anatomy of a relationship

An anatomy of a sequence of movements and a musical score

1 *An Anatomie in Four Quarters* is a visual poem concerned with human beings' insatiable desire to get closer to things, celebrating the physical structure of the bodies we inhabit and the ways we attempt to see, define, contain, name and value them.

2 Bodies seem very different depending on where you are looking at them from – whether that be a particular place in the theatre, a period in history, or your relationship with the person you are looking at.

3 There has always been an intimate connection between anatomy and performance. The anatomy theatre is a kind of 'looking machine' and so is the dance theatre and there is a congruency between the theatres of medicine and of drama, both geographically and intellectually. The celebrated Renaissance theatre designer Inigo Jones also designed the Barber Surgeons' Hall, London, which was used for dissection as well as dancing and entertainment (Sawday, 1995, 76).

4 According to Vitruvius (18–15 BC), an architect's designs must refer to the unquestionable 'perfection' (1914, 74) of the human body's symmetry and proportions. If a building is to create a sense of *eurythmia* – a graceful and agreeable atmosphere – it is essential that it mirror these natural laws of harmony and beauty. This strong structural analogy between anatomy and architecture and the way in which certain modes of 'housing' within the body resemble buildings (an embryo, for instance) gained popularity throughout the Renaissance.

5 In *An Anatomie,* it is the movement of the audience that cuts through or dissects the theatre. The audience get a glimpse of the theatre mechanism and the internal structure, the operational guts – attention is drawn to the lighting rig, the fly tower, the iron, stairways, bridges, balconies and lighting grid.

6 The audience is required to drastically alter their viewing position throughout the piece. This idea of shifting perspective is repeated in the musical and choreographic score, where the same melody or movement sequence is repeated, turned upside down or heard and seen from a different angle.

7 *An Anatomie* draws much of the choreography from anatomical images through history; a curious mixture of the scientific, exquisite, spectacular and cruel.

8 In creating the piece, we were interested in the way an idea of 'the body' may be created by its very representation. Our understanding of anatomy is shaped by the mapping of organs and diseases onto the anatomized body in the seventeenth century; our understanding of neurology in the nineteenth century is mediated through photography; and the flourishing of physiology at the turn

of the twentieth century which has a complex relationship with the development of cinematic technologies. This ever-shifting invention of bodies throughout history is an interesting reminder of how science is incomplete and ever evolving. We were interested in the medical/scientific methods of studying the body, both visually and conceptually; in the beauty but also the real dangers of viewing our bodies in isolation from culture – as machines, as pieces of meat and as vessels for carrying DNA.

9 *An Anatomie* encourages ways of thinking of bodies as connected to the environments they inhabit, invests them with the possibility for change and celebrates them as teetering precariously on the threshold between cradle and grave.

STRUCTURE

<u>Tannoy Announcement:</u>

Ladies and Gentlemen. The House is now Open.

Prelude

The audience is seated high up in the upper circle. The curtains are lit red.

As the houselights go down a married couple are ushered in by torchlight. They are late. The woman is obviously distressed and flustered – anxious that her husband is having an affair – that he is hiding something from her. Throughout the piece they will remain in these seats, and, unlike the audience, are unable to shift their perspective. At times we hear her speaking but it is not clear whether her husband hears her or whether her words are an internal monologue. Anatomy is the separation of parts. These people are going into the throes of their own separation – it is painful and exposing. In some sense she is being flayed.

All of her text (with the exception of the first four lines) comes from the Serbian poet Vasko Popa.

<u>She speaks:</u>

I waited and waited.
Where were you?

We can't see anything from here.
Where were you?
Say something. (Popa, 2011)

Sound of bagpipes. The Red Curtain opens. The first cut.

A dancer enters across the back of the stage. As she turns to walk downstage centre, we know that she is aware of our presence up there in the back of the theatre. The theatre is a looking machine.

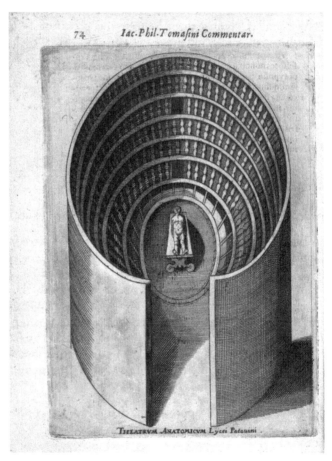

FIGURE 10.1 Theatrum anatomicum lycei Patavini *(1654). Engraving. Image 08652. Image from BIU Santé (Paris), Collection BIU Health Medicine.*

She breathes life into the piece. We see a tiny human body in a big world, her white limbs moving through darkness. Her movement is based on the movement of the lungs. She is like a tree with branches and roots.

First quarter | upper circle

We have a bird's eye view of the tiny figures moving across the stage. The tone is high energy – not frantic but earthbound, celebratory. A kind of evolution takes place – a rising out of the primordial mud. These dancers are flesh and blood; there is no depth, no attention to character or psychology, no clinical angle. We are not being told what to look at and our eyes can wander. The movement language is visceral (tottering, bum dancing, herding, running, spinning and head banging).

In the sound track, we hear an auctioneer at a cattle market bidding. Are these bodies for sale? How much have we paid to watch them? This theme of the value of bodies will reoccur throughout the piece.

In making this first quarter, our visual reference points were medieval imagery of the human body, which shows copulation, pregnancy, birth, old age, dismemberment and disintegration. The medieval body is perpetually transgressing and becoming. It is fluid, contradictory and immeasurable. The medieval image 'ignores the impenetrable surface that closes and limits the body as a separate completed phenomenon' (Bakhtin, 1984, 27). Life and death are viewed as a continuum, death as a liminal space and time. Here human beings are at the mercy of their bodies.

The lights begin to fade on the stage and rise on the couple in the upper circle; the audience is still behind them. He's putting his arm around her, whispering in her ear

She speaks:

> Don't try to seduce me
> I'm not playing
> Don't wind around my legs
> Don't try to entrance me

I'm not coming
My ingenuous breathing
My breathless breathing
Don't try to intoxicate me
I'm not playing
I see
I see
I'm not dreaming
Say something
Say something more
Say something else
Say something different
Say something. (Popa, 2011)

<u>Suddenly, we notice that a dancer has arrived in the upper circle of the auditorium.</u>

She has transgressed the boundaries of the theatre and is now only a few feet away from the audience.

The choreography draws on a selection of sixteenth century *écorché* drawings, where figures, often depicted in the countryside, in nature, are opening their bodies to show the viewer their insides.

Her movements are deliberate and she is aware of our gaze. She is the lover, the femme fatale, a classical, contained, self-conscious figure, unlike the figures we have seen down below. She is an individual, she has agency. She is knowing. She is demonstrating. In much anatomical sculpture and drawing there is a sexual coyness about showing the insides – a woman might be tilting her head, or leaning on her hip as she gazes at the viewer. In the extravagant displays at La Specola Museum, Padua, wax women lie in glass cases with pearls around their necks, wombs exposed.[1]

<u>Lights fade up on stage and there are two figures doing exactly the same movements as the dancer in the auditorium.</u>

We can see the movement at a distance and close up simultaneously. This encourages the audience to be aware of multiple perspectives on a sequence of movements.

The rest of the dancers slowly come back onto stage.

There is a feeling of isolation – the figures are no longer part of an organic whole but shift about the stage as if waiting for something to change. Here, we drew inspiration from Japanese medieval drawings of spirits or *ghaki*. The Buddhist canon repeatedly depicts the ghaki as one 'with a stomach as huge as a mountain but a throat as narrow as a needle'. The somacity of these spirits was the source of their misery (La Fleur, 1990, 272).

It is an unsettled, uncertain place. It is a Space of Possibility. A Betwixt and Between.

Bang!

Lights up.

Again, we see big, bold, organic forms being flung out, with the whole chorus working together. The movement is even more emphatic than before; a reaction to the threat of classical coldness and analysis. The dancers are working together now to demonstrate their solidarity, they cannot be broken apart or analysed away. They are natural, alive, working in harmony, unselfconscious. They are in flux.

Suddenly it goes dark on stage and the lighting gantry directly above the heads of the audience is lit up. We see legs up there doing exercises as if at a ballet barre. They are so close that we can see that they are legs of different shapes and sizes.

We are anatomizing this theatre and its history, and context cannot be disregarded. These balletic bodies are being objectified and truncated, as they have been before, many times, in the history of art.

Lights up on stage

Suddenly, the whole building comes alive, the lighting bars on stage begin moving and different parts of the space are lit up. The structure of the building is being revealed. There are dancers running through the stalls, in the boxes.

Tannoy Announcement:

Ladies and Gentlemen. Please make your way swiftly to the dress circle where you will view the second part of the performance. Please take the nearest available staircase either here or here.

Lights up on hidden internal staircases where access would usually only be granted to technical staff.

The audience cut through the theatre via this privileged route. Everything feels as if it is turning inside out as we begin to get under the skin of the theatre, to go deeper. We are dismantling the house – defamiliarizing it. The audience must take responsibility for their gaze – they can no longer be passive or detached spectators – they must shift their perspective.

The dancers are running, screaming and laughing, the scene has a carnivalesque, Rabelaisian quality. They are throwing off their clothes and doing ridiculous, unsophisticated movements – bouncing, jiggling about and laughing.

By now the audience have arrived in the Dress Circle.

Safely positioned in the best, the most expensive, the most privileged, dignified seats in the house – the scene we are watching on stage seems incongruous from here – messy, wrong, disorganized and embarrassing.

Eleven musicians enter.

They walk across the back of the stage in an ordered line. They are dressed in black suits with white collars – reminiscent of Rembrandt's painting *The Anatomy of Dr Tulp* (1632). They are upright, serious and conscious of the gaze of the audience.

In fifteenth-century Italy, dissection happened at carnival time. There were processional entrances, music and costume. The anatomy theatre was a temple of mortality in which the human form was dismembered.

The musicians cut through the carnival to the front of the stage and as they do so the revelling dancers fall away.

Slowly, over one minute, the front of the stage, with the musicians standing on it, descends (a mechanical pit lift) and we see a light shining from below.

Second quarter | dress circle

We hear the woman. We cannot see her. Her voice is dismembered.

That's better
We've got away from the flesh
Now we will do what we will

Say something
Say something more
Say something else
Say something different
Say something

Someone hides from someone else
Hides under his tongue
The other looks for him under the earth
He hides on his forehead
The other looks for him in the sky
He hides inside his forgetfulness
The other looks for him in the grass
Looks for him looks
There's no place she doesn't look
And looking she loses himself

Why have you swallowed me
I can't see myself anymore
What's wrong with you

Where am I now.

Now no one knows anymore
Who is where, nor who is who
Can you hear me?

I can hear both you and myself (Popa, 2011).

By the time she has finished speaking, the orchestra is in place in the pit. Order has been established. As they tune up their instruments, the black curtain at the back of the stage is lifted to reveal an illuminated white projection screen. It is another cut – a peeling away of the skin of the stage.

In this section, we see projections from *X-ray studies of the joint movements* by John Reynolds (1948).

Projection: FOOT – Effect of the body weight on the arches

This film encourages the audience to reflect on the anatomy of the dancers as they move.

In this second quarter, our visual references for creating material are Classical and Enlightenment. Classical images of the body show a 'finished, completed man, cleansed, as it were, of all the scoriae of birth and development' (Bakhtin, 1984, 25). The messy unfinished nature of pregnancy, birth, old age and death do not fit into the 'aesthetics of the beautiful', as conceived by the late Renaissance, and become secret and removed from sight. The Enlightenment view of the body is as an individualized, discreet object, severed from the material and bodily roots of the world. A strictly completed, finished product, isolated, alone and fenced off from other bodies, self-sufficient and separated from the world. This is the era of uncovering, demonstration, abstraction and epitomization, when the body begins to possess surface, depth and perspective. This 'violent study of depths' (Stafford, 1993, 47) is central to the Enlightenment project and the human body becomes the ultimate visual compendium.

PART 1 Allegro

The musical score is a strict canon, played to an unchanging metronome click. The material is derived directly from melodies found in the first quarter. Here we are looking at the beauty and function of the human body as machine. This section is about scientific method, employed to regularize the messiness and variousness of everyday life. And there is something satisfying about the simplicity of the movement and the predictability of the fugue. The movement is measured. The stage is mapped. We are interested in the *form* rather than the blood and guts. We are happy to be objective. Our gaze is not acknowledged until the last thirty seconds when a dancer wearing a red dress walks onto the stage. Her image appears as a shadow on the projection screen.

<u>Projection</u>: CERVICAL SPINE – Flexion

PART 2 | Largo – Smugglerius

Ten of the dancers are positioned across the stage. Their pose is taken from an *écorché* sculpture known as *Smugglerius* made in 1776 by Agostino Carlini for William Hunter, first Professor of Anatomy at the Royal Academy Schools. The original bronze cast was made from the body of a criminal, thought to be a smuggler, flayed after he was hanged at Tyburn and posed in imitation of the ancient Roman sculpture known as *The Dying Gaul* (see Figure 10.2).

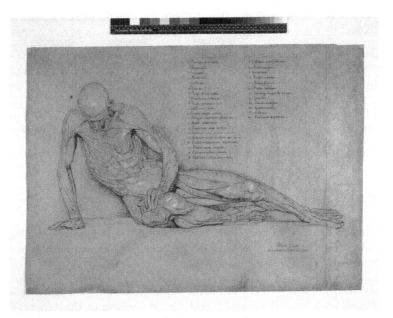

FIGURE 10.2 *William Linnell's* Ecorché *of the 'Dying Gaul' (1840). Drawing. PD.32-1990. © The Fitzwilliam Museum, Cambridge*

Here, the relationship between anatomy and criminality is introduced. The history of anatomical study is rooted in human misery, poverty, punishment and public outrages such as the infamous case of the body snatchers, Burke and Hare.

In terms of criminal punishment, to be anatomized was the ultimate penalty, as it was believed to prevent entrance to heaven. Even in recent history, the relationship between anatomy and criminality prevails. In 1993, Joseph Paul Jernigan, a thirty-eight-year-old Texas murderer was executed and his body cut into 1,871 slices and scanned to become the male cadaver in the Visible Human Project.

<u>Very, very slowly the dancers go through a sequence of movements: they bow their heads, they arch their backs, they drag themselves off.</u>

There is a feeling of shame. Here we are getting a first glimpse of how, from the sixteenth century, interiority became not only a physical but also a psychological state.

<u>All the time the 'Smugglerias' figures are being observed by the dancer in a red dress on the side of the stage.</u>

This is an unashamedly melancholic section – almost romantic – and perhaps the first time we have really thought about death so literally.

Embedded in the score we can hear the voice of a Christie's auctioneer – one million, two million – the price continues to rise.

<u>Projection</u>: SHOULDER – Elevation of Arm.

PART 3 | Allegro

This section continues the investigation of mapping, coding, collecting, classifying, partitioning, controlling, understanding and naming.

At the beginning of this section, the lighting bars descend against the illuminated screen to create a grid. The movement of the dancers is reminiscent of the lines in classical ballet – verticals, diagonals and horizontals. Two of the dancers (in red dress and pink dress) seem to be in control. They are observing the action as if in a laboratory but they are not taking responsibility for the brutality of their gaze. They are detached.

Something darker begins to emerge here and the theme of colonialism and ownership is addressed. In science, especially in medicine, there is a historical idea of 'a necessary inhumanity' (William Hunter, c.1780), which this section questions. We see the humiliation of the specimens. They look like frogs or monkeys in a vivisection laboratory or patients being measured for a study in eugenics. Again, we are reminded that the process of observing alters the thing you are trying to observe – it plays to the gaze.

The specimens leave the stage.

The music ends

We hear a man singing in Italian but cannot see him yet. The remaining 'stage legs' are removed – ghost-like – another stripping back of the layers of the theatre. The stage is completely exposed. We can see the skeleton of the venue.

Tannoy Announcement:

Please make your way downstairs for the third part of the performance. You may sit or stand anywhere in the stalls. Anywhere you like. But be aware of the sight lines of others, as you may be obstructing their view. Thank you.

Lights come up on singing man on the slab.

This is the gruesome price of knowledge, the corpse on the table. This body had a life. He sings. We could even touch him.

In *Birth of the Clinic*, Foucault asserts that at the dawn of western medicine, when the first cadaver was dissected, death left heaven and became the lyrical core of man, 'his invisible truth, his visible secret' (1999, 143).

The words of the song are taken from two sixteenth-century anatomical texts. The words reference Galen's idea of opening up the body in order to see deeper or hidden parts.

Again we hear the woman, she is even further away now.

The myth of Narcissus and Echo is a reoccurring theme in Clod Ensemble's work. Somehow, the woman here is an Echo of sorts – a disembodied voice. In much anatomical drawing an idea of self-reflection and mirroring is present. Anatomia, the 'Goddess of Reduction', is always pictured with both mirror and knife (Sawday, 1995, 3).

She speaks:

> All day you look at your naked reflection in the river of paradise.
> You walk through a whole eternity,
> Along your personal infinity,
> From head to heels and back
> You shine on yourself
> In your head is the Zenith
> In the heels the setting of your shining
> You're walking towards us even today,
> But you can't be seen for shadows.
>
> I plough my face
> It's all I have
> I smash my breasts. What use are they to me? (Popa, 2011)

Third quarter | stalls

Sound of bass guitar, drums

In this quarter, we are drawing from late nineteenth- and twentieth-century images and texts.

This is the most anatomized of the sections, in that sequences of movements and motifs happen simultaneously on stage and do not seem to be connected. Now, we can clearly see the faces of the performers and read their actions in a more psychological way, being encouraged to think of them more as characters.

The themes of cruelty and detachment that were addressed in the final section of the second quarter are played out here. If the first quarter reminded us of the whole body, and the second of the skeleton, this third section is about the viscera, the organs, the mess inside. The internal functioning is echoed in sounds of drums and guitar. There is a visceral brutality about what is happening.

A woman poses on the front of the stage in a swimsuit, compelling the audience to watch as she does the splits.

A woman is being followed, harassed.

A woman is seated on the floor head banging. The dancer in the red dress comes up behind her and tries to force open her eyes.

The lighting bars come down suddenly, and the dancers crouch to avoid their cut. As the bars are pulled out the dancers spring into action in a sequence of movement which takes Francis Bacon's *Painting* (1946) as its point of departure.

A woman runs and leaps into the arms of a man who spins her around and then carries her off – limp, lifeless. There is a suspension here. A moment of transcendence, perhaps.

A woman on stage starts fitting.

Everyone else on stage watches her dispassionately as her movements become exaggerated.

In the nineteenth century, the symptoms of hysteria became exaggerated through the intense relationship between doctors and patients, the viewer and the viewed, the doctor and the diva (Showalter, 1987).

Mass head banging.

A woman tries to map the space as in second quarter.

A woman does a headstand to get a different angle on things but is pushed over.

A group crawls across the stage

It is a strange uncanny choral movement that originally came from thinking about the movement of the head and neck. It feels like they are being forced to do this, as if in an epileptic colony or a concentration camp.

They collapse in a heap of bodies

A woman walks to the front of the stage. She sees the audience and shuts her eyes tight, refusing their gaze. Others surround her, poking and prodding, stretching her legs into seemingly impossible positions. She is lifted up and turned upside down. The soundtrack features traders on the Dutch stock market participating in a voice class to improve their sales technique. They could be trading organs on the black-market.

<u>At the end of the section the company all run to the front of the stage and then to the back wall, as if trying to find an exit.</u>

It is as if they are imprisoned within the walls of the theatre, the body. No way out. The only place to go is in.

<u>Tannoy Announcement</u>

This time the identity of the Tannoy Announcer is revealed and we see the performer in the red dress come out of the wings with a microphone.

Ladies and gentlemen, please come onto the stage. Cut a path through the dancers. Take your time.

Then find a place at the back of the stage. Please be aware of the sightlines of others, as you may be obstructing their view.

Fourth quarter | stage

The audience climbs up the steps onto the stage. They now have an extremely privileged point of view, which would usually be out of bounds to them. The sheer thrill for the audience, of finding themselves on a huge stage, creates a strangeness, an upsetting of the conventional rules of engagement. It is uncanny to contemplate something we know intimately but never see within. An inside outing. The audience perspective has been turned upside down, as they embrace the possibility of looking back on their previous viewing positions.

The chamber orchestra is positioned in the wings. The dancers are repeating many of the movements that we have seen already but deconstructing and reordering them. The audience can see the detail of the movement sequences from close up, see the sweat, the labour, the muscles ripple, hear the breathing. They can make eye contact with the performers. In comparison to where they started it is like looking at the dancers under the microscope.

This section is difficult to describe. Somewhere in it there is a contemporary take on human beings as 'a fold, a crypt, a wrinkle of incidences in the fabric of natures externality' (Pogue Harrison, 1992, 44). Ideas of objective and subjective have collapsed. We see ourselves seeing. Can all viewpoints coexist or be understood at once?

Perhaps, in some sense, at this point in *An Anatomie* we have transcended the authority figure and integrated everything we have learned. In this sense, it is holistic. Even as you are going closer in, there is an opening out – an illusion of depth, infinite complexity and infinite space. The Vanishing Point. The body will always be more than the sum of its parts.

The audience takes new seating positions at the back of the stage. The lights are shining at them so the auditorium seems pitch black. This looking into the darkness, the void, the black hole might induce a state of emptiness, nothingness – a space which induces stage fright or fear of death.

<u>Lights up on the couple, still at the back of the theatre, far away in the distance</u>

As the woman speaks, the dancers repeat the choral crawling movement across the stage. From here, we can hear them try to catch their breath; we can see how difficult the movement is. When they reach the wing, they sit close to the audience and listen.

<u>She speaks</u>

> Give me back my rags
> My raglets of pure dream
> Of silken smiles
> Striped premonition
> And my lace-like sinews
> My raglets of polka-dot hope
> Of filigreed lust
> Calico glances
> And the skin off my face
> Give me back my rags
> I'm asking you nicely

Get out of my walled-in infinity
The dancing ring of stars around my heart
Out of my morsel of sunlight
The rollicking sea of my blood
My flow my ebb
Out of my marooned silence
Get out I said get out
Out of my living pit
…

Get out how long do I have to shout
Out of my head bursting into pieces
Out out just get out

You get childish doll notions
I bathe them in my blood
Dress them in the rags of my skin
Make swings out of my hair for them
Toy carts from my vertebrae
Gliders from my eyebrows
I make them butterflies from my smiles
Wild beasts from my teeth
…
What kind of game is this anyway

I wiped your face off my face
Tore your shadow off my shadow
Leveled the hills within you
Crumpled your plains into hills
Made your seasons quarrel
Kicked the earth's corners from you
Tied the path of my life around you
My overgrown my impossible path
Just try to meet me now

Enough of your sweet-talking immortelles
Of your candied trifles
I don't want to hear to know
Enough enough of everything
I'll say my final enough

Stuff my mouth with earth
Grind my teeth
I'll shut up skull-lapper
Shut up once and for all
I'll stand just as I am
Without root branch or crown
I'll lean on myself
On my own bumps
...
That's all I can do

Don't fool with me freak
You hid a knife under your scarf
Stepped over the line tripped me up
You spoiled the game
You wanted my heavens to turn over
The sun to break my head
My rags to be scattered
Never fool with another freak
Just give back my rags
And I'll give you back yours. (Popa, 2011)

<u>Again, the lighting bars come down cutting the space like a knife.</u>

But, this time, the audience is beneath the bars.

<u>Reprise of the bagpipe music.</u>

<u>We see the first section of the first quarter again.</u>

But, this time, we see the dancers' faces, rather than their backs. There is something joyful in the movement, ecstatic even. We see the first solo again but now the dancer is in front of us, treelike.

We have arrived at the beginning from a new perspective.

The lights gradually fade up on the auditorium and we see the red velvet seats.

The couple has disappeared.

The company of dancers turn to face the auditorium and walk to the edge of the stage.

The curtain descends.

Applause.

The curtain rises and they take a bow.

The iron comes down. It is the final cut.

As it reaches the floor we see a row of feet repeating the ballet steps we saw way up in the gantry.

The huge stage doors are opened, doors that are usually used to shift the scenery in and out of the theatre.

The audience exit through it.

Finally, flushed out of the body of the theatre onto the streets of London.

———

Background and credits

- ❏ Direction and choreography: Suzy Willson
- ❏ Music: Paul Clark
- ❏ Costume: Sarah Blenkinsop
- ❏ Lighting: Hansjörg Schmidt

Movement created with and performed by:

Zoe Bywater, Mariana Camiloti, Valentina Golfieri, Laura de Vos, Silvia Mercuriali, Matthew Morris, Pari Naderi, Ramona Nagabczynska, Yuyu Rau, Ino Riga, Owen Ridley-DeMonick, Alessandra Ruggeri, Sarah Cameron, Jason Thorpe.

Musicians:

James Keane, Nuno Silva, Galen Nikolov, Catherine Ring, Natalia Bonner, Calina de la Mare, Alison Dods, Tom Piggott-Smith, Kate Robinson, Sarah Malcolm, Rebekah Allan, Chris Pitsillides, Chris Allan, Desmond Neysmith, Natalie Raybould

Produced in association with Fuel. A Sadler's Wells commission. Research supported by Jerwood Studio at Sadler's Wells.

Supported by a Wellcome Trust Large Arts Award and Arts Council England.

Anatomie in Four Quarters was first performed at Sadler's Wells Theatre in London, 2011 and adapted for Wales Millenium Centre in 2013.

11

On the Emergent Properties of Death: When Words Fall Apart

Helen Pynor

Foreword

This chapter co-opts a range of voices that circle around the liminality of the life–death border and the inter-subjective borderlands of organ transplantation. These voices are drawn from the biomedical sciences, the humanities and from events and experiences that took place during the making and staging of The Body is a Big Place, *a large-scale immersive installation and performance work exploring organ transplantation made by Peta Clancy and myself between 2010 and 2013.*

*   The Body is a Big Place *re-enacted certain defining aspects of the human heart-transplant process. In performances staged within the installation, a heart perfusion device was used to reanimate, to a beating state, a pair of fresh pig hearts obtained from an abattoir. Rather than sensationalizing these actions we sought to raise questions about the ambiguous status of these disembodied hearts, and to encourage empathic responses from viewers, appealing to their somatic senses and fostering their identification with the hearts they were watching, perhaps opening up a deeper awareness and*

connection with their own interiors. Alongside the heart perfusion device was a five-channel video projection featuring members of an organ transplant community in Melbourne, individuals who had received, donated or stood closely by loved ones as they received or posthumously donated human organs. The video was filmed in a swimming pool where performers repeatedly gathered for a kind of 'meeting'.

In this chapter, my use of disparate and sometimes disjunctive voices reflects my collaborative practice as an artist, in which I borrow scientific and medical methodologies and displace them into cultural contexts where their meaning is radically altered. As an artist whose first training and practice was in science, the practice and language of science feels quite native to me. However, whilst science and medicine seek to achieve a philosophy of certainty that can guide, for example, those deciding at what point it is acceptable to remove organs for donation from a human beating heart cadaver, I am exploring a philosophy of uncertainty. The disjunctive voices I use in this text comment on the relations between art and science, their immiscibility of purpose, and how meaning can nevertheless be generated via their carefully staged, sharp and unapologetic intersections.

Waiting for a heart to start

On May 20, 1999, at 1820 h, an experienced female off-piste skier aged 29 years fell while skiing down a waterfall gully [in Norway]…The woman became wedged between rocks and overlying thick ice, and the space was continuously flooded by icy water…7 min later, her friends called the emergency medical dispatch centre at Narvik Hospital by mobile telephone. The woman struggled under the ice for 40 min. At 1900 h she had stopped moving.

At 1939 h rescue teams arrived. They cut a hole in the ice downstream and removed her from the water, at which time she was clinically dead. Basic CPR was started immediately. An air ambulance arrived at 1956 h…CPR and positive-pressure manual ventilation bag-to-tube was continued during the 1 h flight to Tromsø University Hospital. They arrived at 2110 h.

The patient was immediately taken to the operating room. She had no spontaneous respiration or circulation, her pupils were widely dilated and unresponsive to light. Electrocardiography was isoelectric. Separate electronic pharyngeal and rectal temperature probes measured initial temperature as 14.4°C. An arterial blood sample showed normal serum potassium and oxygenation, moderate hypercarbia, and severe metabolic acidosis.... Foamy pink fluids streamed from the endotracheal tube. A team of cardiac surgeons, anaesthesiologists, perfusionists, and specialised nurses continued CPR...while the patient was prepared for cardiopulmonary bypass by femoral access [assisted heart and lung function]...Systolic arterial blood pressure was around 75 mm Hg measured at a femoral-artery catheter during CPR. Full cardiopulmonary bypass bloodflow was reached at 2150 h. Rectal temperature decreased to 13.7°C at 2152 h. Mean arterial pressure was kept at 50 mm Hg; cardiopulmonary bypass flow started at 0.5 L/min and increased to 3.5 L/min as the venous return improved.

A maximum temperature gradient of 10°C was maintained between the woman's venous blood and the heat exchanger of the cardiopulmonary-bypass machine. At 2200 h, ventricular fibrillation started, which converted spontaneously to a pulse-generating cardiac rhythm after 15 min.

... At follow-up, 5 months after the accident, [the patient] had residual partial pareses [weakness or partial loss of voluntary movement] of the upper and lower extremities that was improving. Her mental function was excellent and she was gradually returning to work. She had also resumed hiking and skiing (Gilbert et al., 2000, 375–6).

Waiting for a heart to stop

At a meeting of intensivists for our benefit at the Baystate ICU [Intensive Care Unit, Baystate Medical Center, Massachusetts, USA], the doctors were discussing non-beating heart cadavers.

'You get the patient declared [dead], and then they try to resuscitate him and take the organs. It doesn't make sense to resuscitate them first', said one doctor.

'What's the difference?' another doctor shot back. 'You're letting a patient arrest and then taking the organs, or you're taking the organs and letting the patient arrest. It's a semantic thing.'

'How long do you wait?' we asked.

'You resuscitate them until you get a [intravenous] line in.'

'You take the patient off his ventilator, wait for his heart to stop, and then resuscitate him?'

'Some don't arrest, and you have to take them back to the ICU or back to a [ward].'

I sensed that some of the doctors were confused (Teresi, 2012, 228–9).

Dying slowly

1

Dying is a process rather than an event. The determination and certification of death indicate that an irrevocable point in the dying process has been reached, not that the process has ended. Determination of death by any means does not guarantee that all bodily functions and cellular activity, including that of brain cells, have ceased. Several tissues can be retrieved for transplantation long after death has been determined by cessation of circulation. Similarly, after death has been determined by loss of whole brain function, the circulation can be maintained for hours or days to enable organs to be retrieved. Maintaining the circulation can continue even longer: for example, in the case of a pregnant woman, so that the foetus can reach viable independent existence (Australian and New Zealand Intensive Care Society, 2010, 12).

2

In 1976, a Conference of the Royal Colleges and Faculties of the United Kingdom published a statement called *Diagnosis of Brain Death*, which set out preconditions and diagnostic criteria for establishing when death had occurred in patients whose vital functions were being maintained mechanically.

In 1979, this statement was supplemented with an opinion in a second statement, called *Diagnosis of Death*, that brain death represents the stage at which a patient becomes truly dead, whether or not the function of some organs, such as a heartbeat, is still maintained by artificial means.

In 1995, the United Kingdom uniquely defined brain death as brain-stem death, being irreversible loss of the capacity for consciousness together with the irreversible loss of the capacity to breathe. This definition is used in some Commonwealth countries but not in Australia or New Zealand (Australian and New Zealand Intensive Care Society, 2010, 11–12).

Irreversible

1

Bernat argues that the Pittsburgh policy [devised in 1993 in Pittsburgh, USA to guide removal of organs from so-called 'non-heart beating donors'] relies on a faulty definition of irreversible. Just because one chooses to not try to restart the heart does not mean it cannot be restarted. Until the heart (or the brain) loses the potential for resuming function, the loss is not irreversible and the patient should not be declared dead (DeVita and Arnold, 2007, 84).

2

Because death, like life, fundamentally is a biological phenomena [sic], determining the definition and criterion of death are biophilosophical tasks that can be studied and modelled but cannot be assigned arbitrarily. Much of the current scientific debate on the coherence of the concept of 'whole brain death' as a formulation of death results from our incomplete understanding of the theoretical biology of complex organisms and their emergent functions. Our current models of complex living systems remain primitive .... But it is from this biological perspective that I hold that my account of the definition and criterion of death best captures the objective reality of the demise of the human organism (Bernat, 2007, 85).

When words fall apart

The body's progress from the end-of-life towards death is illegible. When we use language to arrest the slide we inevitably fall into polarities and binaries, trading uncertainties for certainties and then reversing our position. In the face of death's undecidability language tempts us to contradict ourselves. Rather than the issue getting clouded by semantics, the reverse seems closer to the truth – that semantics get clouded by the issue.

In her book The Body in Pain *(1985), Elaine Scarry discusses the structure of torture and the way language falls apart in its face; inadequate as a means to deal with the body in extreme physical pain. Language can approach the end-of-life (but never arrive) perhaps only by enacting its own breakdown – words sliding down the page or seeping through paper to form slow spreading stains, menacing lumps, senescing meanings and rotting syllables. Falling apart, perhaps absorbed eventually into other bodies.*

Abattoir[1]

1

We're wedged into a corner of the abattoir by a worker with a blow torch scorching hairs off freshly-killed pig carcasses as they move past us on the conveyor belt. The main floor is a soupy mix of water, blood and small pieces of pig tissue streaming steadily towards floor drains. The combined noise of tumbling machinery, the conveyor belt and water jets is deafening and we shout to be heard.

The mass of organs is flung onto the concrete floor at our feet and the pig carcass they came from is inching away from us on the conveyor belt. We scrabble through the warm wet mass but stop when we see the pig's heart, a trembling piece of rhythmic wetness, still beating, and the intestines convulsing in purposeful, peristaltic waves like a pile of slow-moving worms, continuing to digest food that no longer has a body to nourish.

2

Monday afternoon.

Everything goes wrong. Perfusion device not ready. Grumpy and not enjoying this, wishing Peta was here and hanging out for Mike to arrive.

Reschedule from full test of perfusion device to scaled-back dress rehearsal.

Fresh pig's heart and blood put in fridge overnight, next to the lunch boxes of staff from the gallery.

Tuesday afternoon.

Heating system still not ready. Attach heart to perfusion device anyway. Start blood running.

Pose for photographer.

Ignored it at first. Someone else pointed to it.

The resilience of cells.

3

Standing in the small room, with the freshly killed pig carcass hanging from meat hooks suspended from a steel conveyor rack.

The carcass is stripped of skin and innards including the heart we took for our perfusion and it's sliced down the middle.

The flesh hangs there, a mirror image of itself in two halves.

The muscles, bared to us, are a mosaic of twitching restlessness passing in mad waves over the surfaces of themselves.

I'm startled and turn to Gorazd. He says they keep doing this for hours.

Thinking without a brain

1

Imagine a decapitated frog. This frog has lost cerebral control of its body, yet its muscular and peripheral nervous systems function normally: appropriately stimulated, the frog's limbs will move in a manner not unlike that of an intact frog. Imagine now that a drop of acid is placed on the thigh of the decapitated frog. The acid irritates the skin. The headless frog responds to this stimulant in an uncanny manner; employing a behaviour that is routine for a normally functioning frog, it uses the foot on the affected leg to wipe the acid away. Imagine finally that this foot is amputated. The decapitated frog struggles for some time to remove the acid in the same manner (i.e., with its footless leg). Eventually, after reflecting on the fruitlessness of this method, the frog uses the foot on its other leg to successfully rid itself of the aggravating acid.

… A reflex is often considered to be a degraded, nonpsychological form of behaviour, but the frog's behaviour demonstrates otherwise. The truncation of the frog to its reflexive and peripheral substrate reveals anything but rudimentary or mindless action. The frog's peripheral nervous system demonstrates an unexpected intricacy; most pointedly, it seems to have the capacity to respond inventively. Even in this reduced, decerebrated state, the frog's nervous system is thoughtful (Wilson, 2004, 63, 64).

2

Four published prospective studies of cardiac arrest survivors have demonstrated that paradoxically human mind and consciousness may continue to function during cardiac arrest. This is despite the well demonstrated finding that cerebral functioning as measured by electrical activity of the brain ceases during cardiac arrest, thus raising the possibility that human mind and consciousness may continue to function in the absence of brain function.

… The consensus of opinion raised by the authors of these studies has been that the occurrence of lucid well-structured thought processes together with reasoning and memory formation as well as an ability to recall detailed accounts of events from the period of resuscitation is a scientific paradox. This is due to the fact that the studies of cerebral physiology during cardiac arrest have indicated that cerebral blood flow and cerebral function are severely impaired and therefore consciousness would be expected to be lost (Parnia, 2007, 933, 935).

Methodology for retrograde Langendorff perfusion of two porcine hearts

Pig hearts perfusion performance, The Body is a Big Place, Galerija Kapelica, Ljubljana, Slovenia, May 2013.

Abattoir: Two adult Slovenian farm pigs, weighing approximately 70 and 80 kg, were stunned by pistol and exsanguinated by incision of the carotid artery. Fresh blood was collected directly from the carotid incision into a container with heparin (20,000 U) and thereafter stored on crushed ice. The thorax and abdomen were opened and heart removed. The aorta was cut 4 cm distal from its origin and the connective tissue removed. A cannula was inserted into the ascending aorta and the heart infused with 2 L of ice-cold St Thomas' cardioplegic solution at a perfusion pressure of approximately 80 mmHg. Thereafter the hearts were stored in organ bags at 4°C with chilled cardioplegia. Time elapsed from stunning of animal to administration of cardioplegia was approximately three minutes. Pig carcasses from which hearts were removed continued in the food production chain.

Fresh blood and hearts were transported to the gallery.

Gallery: 2 L of perfusate was made for each heart comprising 1.2 L fresh pig blood obtained from the same animal as the heart, 5,000 U heparin, 500 mL Gelofusine (used as oncotic agent) and 300 mL Krebs Henseleit buffer with component concentrations modified to account for diluting effect of the Gelofusine. Major arteries and veins of hearts were trimmed and hearts flushed with tepid Krebs Henseleit buffer then attached to the perfusion system via the aortic cannula. Total time lapse between exsanguination of pig at abattoir and commencement of ex vivo heart perfusion at gallery was approximately sixty minutes.

For each heart a retrograde Langendorff recirculating perfusion system was used, consisting of: roller pump; membrane oxygenator with inbuilt blood filter (pore size 20 μm), membrane oxygenator pumped continuously with carbogen (95% O₂ and 5% CO₂), and heat-exchange system; stand-alone heater-recirculator; and glass heat exchanger placed 35–45 cm above heart.

After connecting hearts to the perfusion system, the perfusate was circulated and the temperature was increased to 37°C over five min. The perfusion pressure was kept constant at 90 mmHg. Upon warming, hearts commenced spontaneous fibrillation and were defibrillated using a single pulse of 200 J at which point hearts commenced beating in sinus rhythm.

One heart was paced for a period of time. Hearts were intermittently stimulated with bolus infusions from stock concentrations of noradrenaline, CaCl₂, KCl, NaHCO₃, glucose, Krebs Henseleit buffer (with adjusted higher concentrations of components as above) and insulin, administered by syringe into the tubing directly above the hearts. After nine hours of continuous beating the heat-exchange and heater-recirculator systems were turned off and the perfusate temperature fell to room temperature (approximately 22°C). Time interval between initial attachment of heart to perfusion system, through to complete cessation of cardiac contractions, was ten hours for heart 1 and twenty hours for heart 2.

Faltering

1

All [potential transplant] patients have a compulsory psychiatric consultation, but they are nowhere alerted to, nor encouraged to reflect on, the half-hidden anxieties and fears that many of them falteringly express with respect to the incorporation of what is essentially an alien organ. All will be told again and again that they will have to take immuno-suppressant drugs for life in order to circumvent rejection, but neither the reality of incorporating the DNA of the other, which will always remain clinically alien, nor the much-reported experience of psychic alterity, is explained (Shildrick, 2008, 16).

As many previous studies have recorded, recipients frequently seek out their donors, or vice versa, (or in the case of cadaveric donation, their families), to claim a kind of kinship. The encounter – if it occurs – may be disturbing for all sorts of reasons and might even amount to a form of harassment. What is clear is that many recipients – in defiance of the objectified machine model – both experience and seek to realise a psychic bond with the other, or their proxies, whom they now feel to be part of themselves. Even in the absence of actual identifying information, the normative divisions between self and other are elided in a highly personalised way (Shildrick, 2008, 17).

2

...the artists [Helen Pynor and Peta Clancy, *The Body is a Big Place*] have worked with members of the transplant community by collectively making an (quite literally) immersive video sequence of a range of humans sharing the same fluid space with one another. This space is represented as a peculiarly social zone – like a waiting room – that becomes untenable, impossible to inhabit from breath to breath. It is a space that all participants cannot share constantly although efforts are continually made to return to the circle of chairs at the bottom of a deep pool of water. In this sense the work goes some way to expressing the complexity of personal and emotional relationships within the transplant network, where relationships are usually anonymous and where, even without anonymity, reciprocation would be an impossibility (Dean, 2011).

3

Overhearing our endless Skype meetings with the underwater videographer, Oron reminds us of the medical dangers inherent to our plan. We ask all participants to get medical clearance but during the long process of home visits to do wardrobe fittings and throughout the gentle conversations that emerge as auditionees traipse back and forth across lounge rooms in ever-new combinations of clothes, these dangers linger at the back of our minds.

In the water we audition the twelve willing participants – organ recipients, tissue donors, and their close family members.

The group has a large team of supporters by the side of the pool, we're struck by the collegiate, generous atmosphere and ponder the impact of being the givers or receivers of such 'gifts' – that burden recipients with knowledge that a death enabled their own ongoing life.

The oldest member in the group has had a lung transplant. She's the one we're most nervous about yet she's desperately keen to make the final cut. But as the audition progresses she, along with roughly half the group, can't manage the demanding task so is left to swell the ranks of the support crew. With Flick's help we hone the remaining swimmers' skills in staying underwater against instincts that command one to rise back to the surface.

We spend a long night at the pool, the group repeatedly sinking to the bottom to commune in a meeting in which something is shared but not words nor barely sight, which become impossible in this environment. Stuart and Flick are the most comfortable in this altered reality and, unplanned, their chairs edge away from the main group until they appear to stage a more personal one-to-one meeting, the rest of the group forming a silent audience to an unknown transaction. By the end of the night we've sent one of the support crew to a late night chemist to find drops for chlorine ravaged eyes, the performers bravely continuing long past the point when common sense would have dictated an end to proceedings.

Later, Peta shows the group footage of the underwater performance and our early tests of the perfused beating pig hearts. Roxanne likens these beating hearts to her own transplanted heart, donated by a dying woman, now firmly lodged in Roxanne's chest – artery to artery, vein to vein. But the vagus nerves of donor and recipient remain unattached, loose ends floating freely in fluid cross currents, this final step of seamless unification remaining forever unfinished.

4

Tammy develops renal failure and Barry donates his left kidney. The doctor says his kidney has a better chance of being accepted in Tammy's body because they have a child together.

The kidney, like a new baby stitched softly into Tammy's flesh.

Cells amass for war, but in the noiseless exchanges of molecular intimacies they remember and forget their differences; the half-whispered murmurs of cellular dreams.

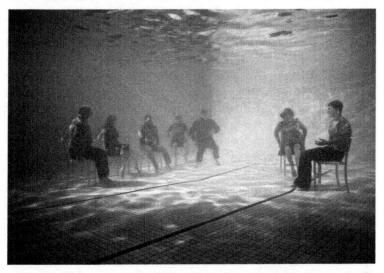

FIGURE 11.1 *Helen Pynor and Peta Clancy,* The Body is a Big Place *(2011) Video production still. Photo by Chris Hamilton. Image courtesy of the artists.*

Fields

1

The experiences of transplant recipients and their donors present a challenge to the notion of the unitary subject and quickly dismantle the self-other binary. Organ transplantation demonstrates the body's passage across vast geographical, temporal and interpersonal distances during the transfer of an organ from one body to another. In this sense, the body is a big place. It is tempting to argue that the disruptive effects of contemporary technologies have enabled this ontological shift but when the body is examined more closely such instances of self-other erasure become commonplace – from pregnancy to the complex ecologies of micro-organisms that co-habit our gastro-intestinal tracts and arguably have profound impacts on our physiological and psychological states. Perhaps technology highlights and extends an already existing propensity for human and non-human bodies to transgress, cross-infect, co-create and fall apart across the borders of organs, individuals, psychologies, species, the cultural domain and time.

The mingling of bodily tissues and resulting hybridity accompanies all forms of medically donated tissue, whether blood donated at a local collection centre, a kidney obtained surgically from a living donor, or vital organs such as hearts and lungs that could only be procured from a cadaveric donor. It is, however, unique to cadaveric donation that the temporal dimension of death is extended, from minutes and hours to years and sometimes decades as a donated organ lives on in the body of a recipient. In this case the dissolution of the self-other binary is accompanied by a second dissolution, that between living-dead. A reading of the body that vests the capacity for 'thought' and consciousness in non-brain tissues adds unfathomable psychic and experiential complexity to the act of organ transfer.

2

Organ donation from cadaveric donors, and new and emerging resuscitation technologies, are both enabled by a liminality inherent to the ontological structure of death. This liminality rests on an existing capacity of cells and tissues to return to health from a point we have arbitrarily designated 'clinical death'. Yet in descriptions in the medical literature and popular media of the chain of collaborative effort lying behind new and remarkable resuscitative feats, unfurled like a magician's silk before a mesmerised audience, it is the biological's pre-existing propensity for resuscitation that (perhaps too obvious to mention) is erased from the narrative.

During the processes of resuscitation and organ transplantation the biological is not a passive or neutral substrate upon which technology acts, but a highly individuated entity with particular histories and capacities. The outcome of any medical intervention articulates the cumulative effects of these bio-personal propensities – the capacities, even the mood, of individual cells and tissues – that collaborate or collide with the bodies and capabilities of clinicians, the technologies they use, and other stochastic and sometimes competing forces to advance a process: a process of multiple and collaborative authorship, an unfolding whose outcomes could never be predicted in advance.

3

... as a critique of binarism, along with deconstruction and other post-structuralisms, a Deleuzian framework poses a striking alternative: rather than the either-or choice imposed by binarisms, they posit a both-and relation. Deleuze and Guattari will readily acknowledge that one must pass by way of or through binaries, not in order to reproduce them but to find terms and modes that befuddle their operations, connections that demonstrate the impossibility of their binarization, terms, relations, and practices that link the binarily opposed terms (Grosz, 1994, 181).

Sinking

1

The hearts beat for ten hours and twenty hours respectively.

Unprepared for this, Peta and I sleep on the gallery floor to watch over them during the night. I sleep fitfully and wake to check them periodically. When we wake in the morning the second one is still beating.

At 1 am the next night after dinner out Gorazd, Peta, Simon and I drive the hearts out of town to a deserted swamp on the Ljubljansko Barje. We bury them in holes we dig into the earth with makeshift shovels and candles bought at a service station on the way and the car headlamps for light.

Damp air, wet grass. An aural cacophony of frog song, hymns for freshly dead hearts.

2

Water is the basic element of the origin and survival of the Barje plain, and at the same time the element, which has been in this area always either lacking or superfluous. At the Barje, water has two different faces. The first is dirty red, stagnant water, slowly trickling from the Barje land. The other is vivacious, pure water of karst origin, flowing from numerous karst springs under Mt. Krim into streams and rivulets, whose last stop at the Barje is the Ljubljanica river. We also call it the river of seven names, for during its course it sinks and reappears on the surface several times, the last time from the springs around Močilnik and Retovje as the Ljubljanica. Once upon a time it flew, as a lowland river with no more than a meter drop from its source to outfall, along numerous meanders which, however, can no longer be seen today (Ljubljansko barje visitor information).

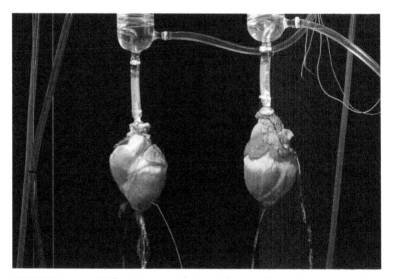

FIGURE 11.2 *Helen Pynor and Peta Clancy,* The Body is a Big Place *(2011) Performance still from live pig heart performance, Performance Space, Sydney. Photo by Geordie Cargill. Image courtesy of the artists.*

Background and credits

The Body is a Big Place

Artists: Helen Pynor and Peta Clancy.
Sound: Gail Priest.

First shown at Performance Space, Sydney in November 2011 and in newly developed forms at Science Gallery Dublin in February 2013 and Galerija Kapelica, Ljubljana, Slovenia in May 2013.

Methodology for pig hearts perfusion performance at Galerija Kapelica, Ljubljana, Slovenia, May 2013:

Collaborating scientist: Dr Gorazd Drevensek, Institute of Pharmacology, University of Ljubljana, Slovenia.
Scientific consultant: Professor Michael Shattock, Cardiovascular Division, King's College London.
Clinical consultants: Dr Kumud Dhital, Dr Arjun Iyer and Jonathan Cropper, St Vincent's Hospital, Sydney, St Vincent's Clinical School – University of New South Wales, Sydney and the Victor Chang Cardiac Research Institute, Sydney.
Curation: Jurij Krpan.

The performance was originally developed for Performance Space, Sydney with collaborating scientists Professor John Headrick and Dr Jason Peart, Heart Foundation Research Centre, Griffith University, Queensland, Australia, and curation by Bec Dean. It was later developed for Science Gallery Dublin with collaborators Professor Michael Shattock, Dr Kumud Dhital, Dr Arjun Iyer and Jonathan Cropper (as above) and curation by Douglas Repetto and Stefan Hutzler.

Early research and development of the performance was undertaken at SymbioticA-Biological Arts, The University of Western Australia, Perth.

(For further details, www.thebodyisabigplace.com)

12

Performing the Microscopic: Beyond Eye and Brain

Alex Mermikides

This chapter examines contemporary performances that seek to represent the microscopic aspects of the human body: those 'objects and functions of the human body that the eye and brain cannot straightforwardly comprehend' (Ede, 2010, 137). The optical comprehension of our bodily interior is not 'straightforward'. As visual historian, Martin Kemp, notes, 'seeing and representing are complex businesses' (2006, 182). Reliance upon an instrument throws into question what Robert Hooke, in his seminal *Micrographia* (1665) calls 'the true appearance' of what lies upon the microscope's stage. Medical technologies that resolve the 'disproportion of the Object to the Organ [the eye]' (in Kemp, 182) offer 'a productively imaginative tool in art and theatre practices that attempt to refocus ways of viewing, and using, bodies' (Parker-Starbuck, 2011, 120). For example, medical images on stage can counter what Devan Stahl calls 'medicine's cold culture of abstraction, objectification and mandated normativity', in which the 'observed body' scrutinized through medical technologies is distanced from the living one (2013, 53). Stahl's account (he is discussing his own MRI scans) follows Cartwright's critique of medical microscopy, in which she suggests that peering through the lens 'effectively distances the observer from the subjective experience of the body imagined' (1995, 83). Liliana Campos argues for the power of theatrical performance to intervene in the objectification of, and 'control' over, the body associated with medical science (in Bartleet and Shepherd-Barr, 2013).

Thus, this enquiry goes beyond the question of how accurately the microscopic might be represented, in order to investigate the emotional responses of an audience confronted with images of its biological minutiae. Performance is here offered as a medium that might 'subjectify' the microscopic, allowing us to somehow 'feel for' cellular components that are visually unfamiliar to a non-expert viewer, and often physically intangible. This is a challenge articulated by artist Helen Pynor as she prepared to embark on a residency at the Max Planck Institute to learn techniques of cell culturing and *in vivo* microscopy. In moving from a focus on whole organs in *The Body is a Big Place* (see Chapter 11), she expressed the concern that while 'it is easy for a viewer to empathise with a heart ... we know what it looks like', cells fall outside of our 'zone of perception': how, she asks, might we bring the cellular 'to presence' and enable a 'visceral, embodied response?' (Pynor, 2014, email correspondence with author).

The chapter collates diverse projects in which the whole body of the performer is displaced or augmented by microscopic anatomies. This disturbance of dramaturgical conventions wherein the (whole) human figure constitutes the main representational vehicle draws me to the current scholarly debates relating to 'post-dramatic', 'alternative' or 'inter-medial' 'science plays'. Shepherd-Barr stakes out this field by defining the 'alternative science play' as one that forgoes the dramaturgical staples of character and narrative in favour of an 'experiential' encounter with science (2006, 201). That said, while Shepherd-Barr's concern is with 'science and *theatre*' (my emphasis), the discussions below also cover dance, interactive digital artwork, bio-art and a public lecture presentation. Thus 'performance' is here defined broadly, as an act of looking at, at least one body, by a live audience in the expectation of some sort of emotional effect. My survey of such projects opens with two sections that trouble Ede's conjoining of 'the eye and brain' as organs for comprehending the body.

The 'Unintelligible' body

What I offer in this first section are two projects that deal with our brain's failure to completely comprehend the body's minute workings, despite advances in medical science that reveal the body at ever increasing levels of magnification. The section reminds us that 'the body' is not a fixed and knowable entity (a point made also by Drew Leder whose *The Absent Body* exposes the impossibility of fully knowing even our own bodies), and that, in some cases, emotional resonance can be found in the body's unintelligibility rather than its intellectual 'comprehension'. The 'unintelligibility' of the body equates with what Vanden Heuvel describes as 'the enigmatic and discontinuous qualities of the postclassical sciences, where crises of visualisation, proof and representation are most apparent' (in Bartleet and Shepherd-Barr, 2013, 367).

Jay Walker's presentation at the *Imagining the Future of Medicine* event at the Royal Albert Hall in London[1] is typical of the TED style of delivery: a head mic. leaves the speakers' hands free for emphatic and well-choreographed gesture; without a lectern, the speaker has free movement across the stage; the earnest delivery carefully orchestrates its rhetoric for maximum audience engagement. The slickness of this presentation is unsurprising given that Walker is founder and chairman of TEDMed. What is unusual, however, is the emphasis it placed on how *little* we know about the human body, in a format that otherwise eulogizes the social impact of scientific discovery, positing the acquisition of knowledge and the innovation of new technologies as the solution to significant human ills. Intended as an introduction to synthetic biologist Paul Freemont, Walker's point was that the human significance of synthetic biology is at least equal to that of evolution, and the industrial and technological revolutions put together. However, for me at least, this point was unintentionally overshadowed, indeed contradicted, by a section which focused on the scarcity of current knowledge about the human body. The force of this short section relied on a combination of surprising fact (e.g. that 'in a quarter of all cases of heart disease, the first sign is death') and memorable analogy (our current knowledge of the human body is equivalent to trying to understand the film *A Wizard of Oz* by looking at one frame). Such statements elicited a palpable sense of surprise in the audience. And I would suggest, unbalanced the TED formula, for the match between the perceived problem (the unknowability of the human body) and the solution (synthetic biology) seemed unlikely, unintentionally imbuing the discussions that followed with an air of hubris.

A very different notion of the 'unintelligible' is posited in my second example, an exploratory project by emerging UK-based dance/film artist Marina Tsartsara. Tsartsara is living with a rare chronic metabolic disease called CPT2 metabolic myopathy that causes episodes of excruciating muscular pain. The condition is unusually 'unknowable', in part because of its rarity and therefore its unfamiliarity to the general population, but also because of its invisibility. For CPT2 manifests no detectable outward symptoms between attacks, and, during them, the pain is diffused through the body, difficult to locate and to quantify. Moreover, the disease is barely detectable by current diagnostic techniques. Very few microscopic images of it exist and the one that Tsartsara was able to locate reveals the effects of the disease (a build-up of fat surrounding muscle cells) rather than the disease itself. One result of this, in the medical context, is that clinicians are unusually reliant on the accounts of their patients for diagnosis and monitoring. However, when I first encountered Tsartsara's work in a showing at the National Hospital for Neurology and Neurosurgery in London (January 2014), she was keen to avoid verbal description of her symptoms or explanation of the disease itself. Instead, her methodology involved a deep focus on her own bodily sensations through techniques such as mind-body centring and cellular meditation, then 'translating' these sensations into choreographic work. Her resistance to what she calls 'objective knowledge', her desire to deactivate the audience's 'intellectual' engagement', can be understood as a way of reclaiming control of the body from the medical gaze and of prompting an embodied response in her audience. However, its effect was to produce audience responses that were strikingly dependent upon prior medical knowledge.

For example, in audience discussions following the showing, Tsartsara's neurological consultant described one sketch – in which Tsartsara cranes her head back in order to view a screen showing images of white powder – as 'calming', while, as a non-expert viewer, I described the same scene as 'uncomfortable'. The consultant explained that, while watching Tsartara's other, more energetic, dances made her 'nervous' (physical exertion can trigger an episode), she was reassured when she stood still. The white power, which I viewed as sinister (suggesting cocaine), was understood by the consultant to be glucose powder, administration of which can ward off an attack. The consultant was clearly profoundly moved by the work, whereas, while I admired the project that Tsartsara set herself, it was the neurologist's rather than the artist's description of the disease ('like the day after running a marathon without training – times a hundred') that produced in me the strongest sense of empathetic engagement. Thus, differences in prior knowledge led to almost opposing interpretations of the same performance, and, I felt, absence of this medical knowledge produced a less powerfully sensed empathic response to the material.[2]

Vanden Heuvel's argument, touched on above, is that the appropriate response to the 'unintelligibility' of post-classical science is not 'conventional science plays', but those designed to incite the condition of wonder. He cites Emily Dickinson's poem to describe this as:

> not precisely Knowing
> And not precisely Knowing not
> A beautiful but bleak condition. (in Bartleet and Shepherd-Barr, 371)

The projects examined above navigate this line between 'knowing' and 'knowing not' and as a result produce effects upon the spectator that are beautiful, bleak or otherwise. Moreover, they reveal that understanding does not necessarily result in emotional or empathetic engagement. In Walker's presentation, this came with knowing how little we know. In Tsartsara's, though, the difference between 'knowing not' and 'knowing' exposed a limit to at least one audience member's empathetic response.

The (Im)Permeable body

In *The Transparent Body*, Van Dijck describes the 'endoscopic gaze', a trope commonly used in science-fiction cinema, that zooms into a character's microscopic interior, in an effort to 'get past the physiological borders of the body, the organ, the molecule' and 'surpass the limits of representation' (2005, 79). Van Dijck's example is the 1966 film *Fantastic Voyage*, but the device recurs in more recent screen projects, for example, in episodes of American detective series *CSI* (as discussed by Kuppers, 2007, 164–72), in the spider bite that gives Peter Parker his amazing powers in Sam Raimi's *Spider Man* (2002) and, as a mild spoof, in a snail that is endowed with great speed in an encounter with a race car in Dreamwork's *Turbo* (2013). For live performance, of course, the 'limits of representation' are more difficult to surpass than through the computer-generated imagery available to screen. In this section I consider productions that seek to emulate the 'endoscopic gaze' but ultimately foreground the struggle for live performance to transcend the skin boundary of the body. Thus, while the focus in the section above was on what the 'brain' cannot straightforwardly comprehend, here I turn our attention to the limits of the 'eye'.

Jean Abreu's *Blood* (2013–2014)[3] is described on the maker's website as 'one man's scientific exploration of his flesh and blood that leads him in search of the composition of his soul'. In this solo show, the 'zoom' is two-way, both exteriorizing and interiorizing. Purportedly choreographed 'from the inside out' (Winship, 2013), Abreu seeks to externalize what he can of the bodily interior, producing and exploring spit, sweat and urine. His movements (amplified through a reactive videoscape featuring a digital body double and images of bodily fluids from Gilbert and George's *Fundamental Pictures,* a series of pictures based on microscope slides of body fluids) nag at his own skin to discern what lies beneath: he tests his own pulse, traces his blood vessels, administers knee taps, reaches into his mouth and drinks water. Ultimately, though, what is staged here is the impossibility of transgressing the surface boundary, of zooming more than a few inches out, a few millimetres in: we remain firmly at a distance, the projected microscope images exposing Abreu's, and our own, failure to see inside. The production, according to reviewer Sarah Wilkinson, depends on what she calls an 'objective intimacy' towards the body: 'something so recognisable and personal…made unrecognisable and strange' (2013). Other reviews also alluded to this 'objective' orientation, but as an undesirable sense of detachment: the production, according to Jan Parry is 'impersonal' (2013).

A stronger sense of engagement is produced by an interactive digital artwork entitled, *The Primary Intimacy of Being* (2014). This is composed of a large screen which acts as a full-body mirror to the viewer. Standing at a distance before it, the viewer sees a glowing outline of what appears to be her own body. Moving in front of the 'mirror' produces colourful 'trails' that track her gestures and path. As she approaches the screen, her bones, muscles and organs become visible, as if through MRI imaging. Again a sense of 'objective intimacy' is intended: the project website claims that 'a new intimacy is established with the stranger that is our own body' (Maître, 2013).[4] Indeed, research by Xavier Maître into audience's responses to the project, notes some strong, occasionally comic, responses as when a female viewer instinctively covered her bosom to prevent others seeing the 'naked' body of her digital reflection (Griffith, 2014). The strength of such reactions is all the more surprising given that the project employs medical images (which, as noted below, are elsewhere deemed to crystallize the detachment and objectification of the medical gaze), that are static (thereby exposing the artifice of the mechanism) – and, indeed, that the scans used are not, in fact, of the actual viewer. The latter is a practical necessity as it would be impossible to produce such detailed scans in real time, but one that buys into medical science's de-individualization of the body. Descriptions of the project in the popular press make no secret about this device, indeed the technologies employed are prioritized in such accounts and in the project website (it was exhibited in digital technology events rather than arts contexts). This foregrounding of the technology is significant, I would suggest, for while the 'mirror' does not allow the viewer to see to the microscopic level, we are left with the impression that we soon could: the limits, it seems to be saying, are only technological.

Of course, other performance practice transgresses the skin boundary much more radically than these projects, notably in work by ORLAN (especially in her 1990s surgery performances), Franko B and Ron Athey. As Gallego argues in relation to Athey's work, this adoption of the 'dissector's cut' can effect an 'alternation of the symbolic order' (Gallego, 2014, 74). In both my examples above, the permeation of the skin is relatively safe: for Abreu it occurs through 'natural' orifices (the mouth, the urethra) rather than breaching the skin; for Maître, the magnetic field and radio waves that create the images are not only harmless, but also have occurred in another person's body. And the bodily interior is presented as clean, rather than messy or abject: even Abreu's urine is contained in a plastic bottle, the images of body fluids are aestheticized by Gilbert and George's stained-glass colours; bones and organs of Maître's piece are ghostly blue or in primary colours the evoke the aura of photography. However, it could be argued that in both body art and the safer practices discussed here, we are left with the similar result – a failure to fully see, as well as to understand, what is revealed, without this necessarily limiting the emotional engagement with what the 'brain and eye' cannot entirely comprehend.

In the following sections, I discuss two further strategies for bringing the microscopic into the 'zone of perception': the inclusion of medical images within theatrical performance, and the use of anthropomorphic analogy in two examples of bio-art. In both cases, the emphasis is upon the way in which technological mediation is employed to 'subjectify' the bodily components on display.

Subjectifying the medical image

This section offers an exception to Cartwright (1995) and to Stahl's (2013) conception of medical imaging as the crystallization of the objectifying medical gaze, arguing that, in one case at least, medical images provide a means of both intellectually and emotionally bridging the gap between subjectivity and objective knowledge. Here Anna Furse refers to medical imaging associated with assisted reproductive processes (ART): 'imaging technology feeds the imagination, makes what would be invisible to the naked eye have form and shape. It connects us to parts of ourselves at a cellular level, vividly and beguilingly' (Furse, 2006, 163). Images of gametes (sperm and egg), pre-embryos and embryos, as well as the more familiar scans of foetuses, are capable of provoking extremely emotive responses, even at the level of individual cells. Gametes, particularly the tadpole form of the sperm cell, are more readily identified as bodily components than say, skin or muscle cells. Once an ovum is fertilized it becomes a potential person, and for the parents, a much longed for child: 'its image becomes a talisman, a pre-figurative icon of what might evolve to a baby' (Furse, 2006, 163). Thus the 'humanity' (potential or otherwise) of even just a few developing cells can evoke parental protectiveness, ownership, wonder. In this specific realm, emotional engagement with the microscopic is extremely potent.

Here I consider medical images displayed within the stage space that act as a sort of 'window' into *in vitro* biomedical procedures normally unavailable to the naked and non-expert eye. This 'window' may be subsumed within a naturalistic framing, or may be interwoven more poetically within the performance. My first example, a moment in Carl Djerassi's *Immaculate Misconception* (2002) illustrates the former. In scene 5 (which I saw presented by Djerassi himself at the *Performing Science* conference in Lincoln 2014), we witness the protagonist Melanie fertilize an ova (her own) with a single sperm cell (taken, without his knowledge, from her lover).[5] The procedure is enlarged and screened for the benefit of her colleague Felix, and for the audience. We see her pipette suck in the sperm, then inject it into the ova. My second example is Athletes of the Heart's *Yerma's Eggs*, directed by Anna Furse (2003). In this production, the images are less naturalistically employed. Rather than solely representing narrative events, electron microscope images of ova at various stages of conception, similar footage of an ICSI procedure and 3-D scan of a foetus, become expressive of the characters' imaginings, desires and fears; not contained within a screen, but landing on bodies, floor, theatrical grid and fabric held by the performers.

Despite the fact that these two productions deal with similar territory, and indeed, include films of the same procedure of an ovum being fertilized with a single sperm (ICSI), the emotional resonance provoked by the incorporation of these 'windows' into the microscopic is very different. As the brief description above may suggest, the fertilization scene in Djerassi's play raises ethical, social and personal issues: questions of consent and 'ownership' are clearly foregrounded, for example, as is that of a woman's 'right' to motherhood. However, while these are no doubt emotive issues, my experience of this scene was that the emotions evoked by the projected image, occurred in spite of, rather than because of this fictional framing. For example, here Melanie reveals to Felix that the egg that has just been fertilized is her own: 'Why couldn't these eggs *(Points to the microscope)* come from here? (*Gestures toward her lap*). What you saw on this screen came from me' (Djerassi, 1998). However, her words and gesture in fact remind us that these are images from someone else's procedure (the play text attributes this procedure to Dr Pedersen in San Francisco, though the woman and potential child whose images feature so prominently are unacknowledged). The inclusion of film footage of actual procedures emphasizes the topicality of Djerassi's play but simultaneously exposes its fictionality. In Furse's play, by contrast, the images stand for not only the parental desires or memories of its fictional characters, but also those of the performers and the director herself, who all have personal experience of ART (this is made clear in the performance itself and in its publicity material). Director Furse' own daughter, born of IVF, has the last word in the production as her recorded voice describes her conception. The effect of this blending of life and art – reflected perhaps in the pervasiveness of the medical images that are not contained in a screen – adds to the visceral 'subjectification' of the medical images and the power of the performance. In both productions, these 'windows', then, represent a sort of truth claim that punctures the fictional frame of the performance – purposefully, in the case of Furse's play, or inadvertently, in relation to Djerassi's.

Analogy and anthropomorphism

Kemp's discussion of Hooke notes that 'the revealed appearances of things of the minute world in his microscope rely repeatedly on the use of analogies with the familiar world of objects visible to the naked eye' (2006, 183). What I consider here is two bio-artworks wherein an analogy is made between cell cultures and more familiar – indeed, more clearly 'human' (at least to the non-expert eye) – entities. Both works were shown at the Visceral Exhibition in the Science Gallery, Dublin (2011), a tenth anniversary retrospective of SymbioticA projects involving living biological material.[6] The exhibition title is relevant to the concern of this chapter, referring not only to the fact that the works on display come from the body, but also that they are designed to provoke a 'gut feeling in the way people respond when they are being confronted by something that is contradictory to what they perceive life to be' (co-curator Oran Catts in exhibition film[7]).

Like several of their works, Ionat Zurr and Oron Catts' *Semi-Living Worry Dolls* (2000) employs a process of seeding degradable polymer structures with cell cultures to produce 'living sculptures' in shapes that have a stated thematic resonance with the materials and procedures employed in their making. This work draws on the Guatemalan tradition of giving children dolls with which they can share their worries, each of the seven dolls represents an anxiety surrounding tissue engineering (Dublin Science Gallery n.d.). However, I would argue that the doll form is significant to the emotional impact of the work for additional reasons. Chief among these is the fact that the tiny and fragile figures resemble not just hand-crafted dolls, but also children. We read their faces for emotion of their own, endowing them with subjectivity. This anthropomorphic effect is reinforced by the emphasis placed upon them as 'living' (albeit in a 'semi' alive state): as discussed by Sally Jane Norman the presence of their life-supporting bioreactors,[8] through which they are fed and sustained at optimal temperature is a constant reminder (in Bleeker, 2008, 191). Additionally, we are encouraged to confide in them, sharing our own worries either through a microphone set up for this purpose or by sending an email. Zurr suggests that over the course of the exhibition, viewers were liable to 'form some relationship with them': the disposal of the cells at the end of the exhibition evoked deep emotion despite the fact that 'we kill more cells brushing our teeth' (Zurr in exhibition film). Overall, the emotional impact of this work is distinct, I believe, to that evoked by the artists' other bio-sculptures such as the more whimsical *Pigs Wings* (2000–2001) or even the uncanny creation of body parts such as their 2007 work with Stelarc, *Extra Ear ¼ Scale* and *Ear on Arm*.

A similar, if differently inflected, anthropomorphic effect is evoked by Kathy High's *Blood Wars* (2010).[9] This project took the form of a tournament, running throughout the exhibition, comprised of matches that pitched colour-coded white blood cells from different anonymous donors against each other. The matches were filmed through high resolution micro-cinematography that recorded as one person's system eventually destroyed the other's. These 'games' were replayed at high speed during the exhibition.

The tournament form, familiar from sports and games, emphasizes conflict and competition. Indeed, in conceiving the project, High drew on associations of military warfare often attributed to the immune system (High, 2011[10]). What is particularly interesting about the analogy the project makes between human competitive activity (sports and war) and immunological processes is that it equates to the conflict that lies at the heart of Aristotelian dramaturgies. Indeed it echoes David Mamet's notion of theatrical structure as 'the perfect ball-game' (1999, 1–11). Emotional engagement for the viewer, in this example, involves taking sides, sharing in the glory or defeat of the 'competitor' we choose to champion. We are brought, then, to ideas of character: although the blood is provided by anonymous donors, High provides competitor profiles, giving us just enough information to build a character. What is unexpected about both of these projects, then, is that although they are situated in avant-garde and experimental arts practice, they operate through the dramaturgical staples of character and narrative. Thus, the complex processes of the immune response are rendered 'intelligible' through analogy to human scale activities – war, sport and theatrical performance.

Conclusion

In drawing to a conclusion, I focus on two general principles that emerge from these discussions: firstly, the unexpected recourse to the 'dramaturgical staples' of character and narrative noted in relation to the Visceral projects and, secondly, the disturbance of theatrical illusion discussed in relation to Djerassi's work, which also plays out in other examples. I draw upon these principles rather than others raised by the discussions, in part because they represent the tension alluded to in the introduction, between the 'dramatic' and 'post-dramatic' orientations of contemporary science-engaged performance. And because they elucidate how performance practices might allow us to 'feel for' our bodies at a cellular scale.

Our empathy, it seems, continues to be drawn to performers (human or otherwise) that are 'human shaped', rather than cellular or cytogenetic: thus bringing our minute components into our 'zone of perception' requires not only magnification but also a degree of anthropomorphism. There is some leniency here for we can empathize with the almost human (Catts' and Zurr's dolls); the potentially human (the gametes and pre-embryos in Djerassi and Furse); and implied humans (the blood donors outlined by High's 'Competitor Profiles'). A useful parallel might be the tradition of puppetry where only minimal animal characteristics (e.g. eyes and movement) are required to endow an inanimate object with subjectivity. As in puppetry, these human 'shapes', which we might also call characters, are rendered all the more empathetic when they are acted upon, when they seem to suffer: for example, the prick of concern we experience as the needle penetrates the ovum in Djerassi's piece. To this extent, even work that initially seems to lie outside of the 'classic Aristotelian model' draws on fundamental tenets of this tradition: a humanoid protagonist struggling against forces of opposition.

Another surprising discovery is that this dramatic personification is employed irrespective of the particular technologies employed: cell cultures, magnified images of cells and organs, or more abstracted representations of the microscopic. In all cases, bringing our microscopic interior landscapes into the 'zone of perception' requires a degree of mediation: actual cells are made into representations. Moreover, as representations simultaneously take on the resonance of the real, a number of these projects disturb easy binaries that oppose the 'objective' domain of the medical and its engagement with the 'real', with the 'subjective' one of the fictional arts. Indeed, some of the most affecting moments within the performances examined here involved disturbances to theatrical illusion, that is, deliberate or unintentional interruptions to the way that the performing body has been arranged for display. These include the uncanny endowing of subjectivity to living yet inanimate objects in *Semi-Living Worry Dolls*; the allusion to its performers' autobiographic connection to the subject matter in *Yerma's Eggs*; and the unintended, but equally disturbing, claim that Djerassi's fictional Melanie makes upon an ova that, we know, belongs to someone in the real world. The effect in these cases, is often more 'embodied' than empathetic: the vertiginous feeling of having our sense of 'reality' (albeit a fictional one) reframed.

We return, then, to Vanden Heuvel's argument that the 'wonder' evoked by recent scientific discovery is best served by performance that places its audience in a 'position of indeterminacy and instability in relation to how information is processed' (2013, 374). It is all the more appropriate that such performances shift attention from the performing body to that of the audience member – their sensory processes and consequent meaning-making for Vanden Heuvel, or Zurr's idea of the 'gut reaction'. Thus, while for Campos, theatre is 'embodied' because it refracts meaning through the human figure, its deportment and behaviour in relation to others, emerging forms of science-engaged performance might also prompt the audience member to bring their own body to consciousness. In doing so, performance might play a key role not only in reflecting but also in negotiating the profound shifts in our understanding of what it means to be human.

13

Copy, Cut, Paste – Humans (Re-)Printed: Lynn Hershman Leeson's *The Infinity Engine*

Gabriella Giannachi

This chapter is the first study of Lynn Hershman Leeson's *The Infinity Engine* (2014–), an installation that, along with a film of the same name, makes up a hybrid media artwork exploring 'possibilities for evolution now that DNA can be programmed' (Hershman Leeson, 2013a). The work utilizes emerging ideas in communication technology, medicine and biological technology, and draws from cultural studies of identity, including history of science, cyborg theory, feminism, performance, art and fiction. At once time-based installation, film, experiment, evidence and live archive, *The Infinity Engine* installation represents an emerging cultural form situated between science and art, which problematizes the very notion of what constitutes *life* in art and society today, operating beyond the postmodern as a form of 'organic performance'. The defining features of 'organic performance' are presented here as a framework, which extends and challenges Ihab Hassan's well-known table of modern and postmodern dichotomies (1982, 269) in order to reflect new concepts of the human in an age of ground-breaking technological and medical innovation. The framework shows that organic performance, which addresses what constitutes life itself, draws on performative, theatrical and scientific discourses and practices, placing the public as participant and witness to the production of knowledge about what constitutes liveness through laboratory experimentation.

Prologue: The 'copy-cut-paste' body

Hershman Leeson, who is known for her work as a photographer, performance artist, new media artist and documentary maker, has long been investigating the malleability of the body and the fabrication of identity through technology. Thus, for example, her well-known work *Roberta Breitmore* (1974–1978), which combines photo, video and performance, sees Hershman Leeson enact, by wearing a wig, a costume, and make up, the signs of a 'physical embodiment' through 'a set of individual gestures, needs and fears' (Rötzer, in Schwarz and Shaw, 1996, 136). The 'private performance of a simulated persona', Roberta, was thus 'at once artificial and real' (Hershman Leeson, 1996, 330), met only as mediated 'evidence' of past activity over whose veracity, significance and connection the viewer or reader was invited to speculate. These process-driven aesthetic strategies were also significant for her cyborg pieces where, she indicates, it was important to 'see gearshifts and things coming out of [the cyborgs'] bodies' so that 'the mechanics and process of living and being alive' would be exposed. These works, typically for Hershman Leeson, aimed at 'looking at the inside of things, letting the process show' (in Giannachi, 2010, 232), thus already implicitly showing the technological properties of the cyborg body through a medical, even surgical (copy-cut-paste), lens.

As well as being an installation, *The Infinity Engine* also constitutes the concluding part of a film trilogy that includes *Conceiving Ada* (1997) and *Teknolust* (2002). All three feature Tilda Swinton and explore 'the implications – ethical as well as social – of the impact on the human species in an era of genetic manipulation' (Hershman Leeson, 2013a). The trilogy is centred on the theme of the cyborg, the 'self-regulating human machine system[s]' (Featherstone and Burrows, 1995, 2) that has been challenging traditional binaries between natural and human-made entities, leading to the often disputed theorization of the post-human (Gray, 2002). Thus *Conceiving Ada*, using a virtual set composed of 375 photos of bed and breakfast hotels in San Francisco that had a 'Victorian feel' (in Tromble and Hershman Leeson, 2005, 97), features the computer scientist Emmy Coer who, obsessed with Countess Ada Lovelace, the author of the first computer algorithm written for Charles Babbage's Difference Engine, attempts to bring her into the present. Whilst the two women succeed in communicating, they find that gender is a major concern since, unlike Babbage, Lovelace's name is largely forgotten.

The second film in the sequel, *Teknolust*, features the biogeneticist Rosetta Stone injecting her own DNA into a computer programme that generates three self-replicating automata (SRAs), named Ruby, Marine and Olive, after the red, green and blue pixels used to create colour on the computer monitors, that grow on her computer. These need to adventure into the real world to receive the Y chromosome that keeps them alive. To achieve this, Ruby is programmed to absorb images from films so she can re-enact love scenes in real life, meet partners, collect their semen and share it with the other two automata – though the men she meets appear to develop a strange disease. Subsequently, the three pursue their own adventures: Ruby develops an encrypted language that allows her to talk to her sisters in secret; Olive reads psychology, philosophy and history texts; and Marine hacks into Rosetta's computer to steal her code for the cloning. In the end, Ruby falls in love with Sandy, a print shop employee, and has a child with him. For Jackie Stacey, the three digital clones embody a tension between sameness and difference. As cyborgs, she suggests, they are a combination of genetic and computational material, both human and non-human, single and multiple, and emerge from a culture of coping that is digital and genetic (Stacey, 2010), technological and medical.

The third film in the trilogy, *The Infinity Engine*, features Iris, who is seen as a nineteen-year-old coming to terms with being 'the first human to have received a bio printed heart and the tenuous nature of her life' (Hershman Leeson, interview with Giannachi, 2014). In this case, Tilda Swinton takes on the role of a glowing rebel cat – glowing because she carries the genetic code of a jellyfish, the green fluorescent protein (GFP). Her character searches for freedom, enlightenment and the company of humans in a biotechnology company. The choice of the cat was inspired by the green glowing cats that had been injected with the GFP which were created by researcher Eric Poeschla at the Mayo Clinic in Rochester, Minnesota in 2011 for the study of the feline immunodeficiency virus, which played a crucial role in building an understanding of HIV/Aids.

Parode: The replicating body

Hershman Leeson's artworks are often inter-related and could be described as emerging from one another. Thus *Roberta Breitmore* bred out from *The Dante Hotel* (1993), a site-specific installation set in the run-down Dante Hotel on Columbus Avenue in which visitors encountered an empty room with signs of the presence of a hotel guest who was, however, not physically present in the room. Roberta Breitmore too, one year later, started her 'life' at the Hotel Dante, after stepping out of a Greyhound bus with only $1,800. *Agent Ruby* (2002), on the other hand, bred out of *Teknolust*. In *Agent Ruby*, users log into 'Ruby's E-Dream Portal', also featured in *Teknolust*, from which Ruby can invite them to ask her anything so that she may teach them to dream. If visitors type a question, Ruby then types a response and the conversation begins. Ruby can remember users' questions and names, and she has moods that depend as to whether she enjoyed their company. In a more recent version (2004), Ruby can also respond verbally and can be downloaded to Palm handheld computers from the website. For Hershman Leeson, 'this Tamagotchi-like creature is an internet-bred construction of identity that develops through cumulative virtual use, reflecting the global choices of internet users'. The piece thus, for Hershman Leeson, 'evokes questions about the potential of networked consciousness, identity, corruption, redemption, and interaction' (in Tromble and Hershman Leeson, 2005, 98). All these works, though free-standing, and utilizing different media, take place in a network of inter-related locations, share elements stemming from their plot or story, and feature characters that appear to be related to or even emergent from one another.

Hershman's exploration of symbiosis and replication of the post-human body is significant towards building an understanding of the operation of the organic performance framework used in *The Infinity Engine*. We know that the post-human body is defined by 'symbiotic interdependence', which means that it is characterized by the 'co-presence of different elements, from different stages of evolution: like inhabiting different time-zones simultaneously' (Braidotti, 2002, 226). One of the ways in which this manifests itself in Hershman Leeson's work is the co-presence of works that are related, but interdependent from one another, whose 'liveness' therefore is not a consequence of the time of the execution of the work, but rather of its persistence and generative legacy. We also know that the post-human body tends to be 'viral' or 'parasitic' (Shaviro, 1995). In Hershman Leeson's work, the post-human body is frequently represented through the meeting of the signs drawn from a number of disciplines, which, intertextually, also draw from the aesthetics of works spanning different periods in time. In other words, these post-human bodies are not only in a viral relationship with each other, they are also in a parasitic relationship with other 'bodies' of work.

This ability of the work to replicate (*The Infinity Engine* itself is a replica of a laboratory of science) is not unconnected to what Jean Baudrillard described in relation to the simulacrum, which, for him, duplicates without any pretension of originality (1983). Caught in a cycle of 'successive phases of the image' (Baudrillard, 1983, 11), for Baudrillard, the post-human body is always also 'capital' or 'consumer object' (1998, 129). Except in Hershman Leeson's work post-human replicas maintain an identity, presence even, that makes them distinct from one another. Here, the post-human body, whilst being in a symbiotic relationship with other bodies and possibly replicating aspects of them, remains a subject. This ability to establish their presence is also what makes them persistent. Furthermore, the 'body' of work, that is, Hershman Leeson's opus, mimics this behaviour of the post-human body. It is a consumer object (product), as well as a producing mechanism (process), growing from the inside out, whose capital consists mainly of its generative power (primarily, but not exclusively, established through replication often also occurring via documentation). What therefore emerges from this process is a simulacrum that may not have the substance and qualities of an original, but is nevertheless capable of creating its own 'reality' from which its presence and originality are dependent. Thus, in Hershman Leeson's work, every replica, every copy, can become again an original, with a distinct aesthetic, political and economic value. Additionally, in *The Infinity*

Engine, addressing advances in regenerative medicine through 3D printing, copies are in effect the live prints of our cells, organisms without a body, potentially part of us.

Episode: The readymade body

The Infinity Engine installation consists of the eight-room replica of a genetics lab that is shown in museums and science laboratories. Constructed from modular units utilized in current genetic research, the lab, turned into an exhibition space, includes video interviews with leading experts in genomics, medicine and history of science; performances; photography and experimentation about regenerative medicine, bio-printing, genetically modified organisms and DNA re-programming. Visitors enter the installation via a replica of a genetics lab door. To the right of this, they can enter a black room where the scaffolding of a nose is exhibited. The latter was donated by Wake Forest Center for Regenerative Medicine, specialized at engineering laboratory-grown organs that are successfully implanted in humans. Music playing in this room consists of 'DNA components'. Here is the first 3D printer, which was donated by Organovo, a company designing functional human tissue (Hershman Leeson, 2014a). In the 'anti-chamber', video interviews show Dr Antony Atala, Professor in Regenerative Medicine at Wake Forest, demonstrating 3D bio-printing techniques, and a recipient, Luke Masala, talking about what it means to have one of the first bio-printed organs. In the 'hybridity room', visitors can see wallpaper of genetically modified plants and animals, which are juxtaposed against pictures of labs conducting scientific experiments. A number of iPads are available here so that visitors can see 'the consequences of actions by experts, such as Dr Drew Endy, Professor of Microbiology at Stanford University; Dr Elizabeth Blackburn; and Dr Anthony Atala' (Hershman Leeson, 2014a). In the 'ethics room', file boxes of court cases relating to gene patents are available and cases are discussed by experts such as Dr Myles Jackson, Chair, History of Science, New York University; Dr Troy Duster, Professor Emeritus in Sociology, University of New York; and Andrew Hessel, a futurist and catalyst in biological technologies. At the 'biometric soul catcher installation', visitors can enter data into a visualization that will result in a downloadable live archive. Visitors are captured by a scan that then 'reverse-engenders their facial structure to reveal origins. This becomes part of a mutating but individually retrievable image that can converse about genetics' (Hershman Leeson, interview with Giannachi, 2014). The image visualization also 'allows for DNA input' (Giannachi, 2014). Finally, in the hallways, formed by mirrors reflecting the different lab surroundings seen in *The Infinity Engine*, visitors encounter replicas of lab paraphernalia. The prototype for the work was first seen by the public at the Yerba Buena Center for the Arts in San Francisco in 2013 and the full exhibition opened at the ZKM | Center in Karlsruhe in December 2014.

For Hershman Leeson, the lab 'enacts narratives of a not-too-distant future'. Here, 'organs can be manufactured and banked, lost limbs can be regenerated from the inside out, skin can be printed on an ink jet printer and human life can be extended to 130 years' (2013b). Visitors to the lab, whose images are reflected 'to infinity' in what looks like a wall of mirrors, can directly participate in the work with their DNA, which results in an online cumulative 'intelligent being', 'a constantly mutated archive for all participants who will become an expert on genetic information' (Giannachi, 2014). Through interviews with scientists conducted by Hershman Leeson, we learn about the latest advances in reproductive medicine. Thus, for example, in the interview with Dr Elizabeth Blackburn, Professor at University of California, we learn about her work in telomere isolation, a DNA protecting structure at the end of chromosomes, for which Blackburn won the Nobel Prize in 2009. In analysing the role of telomerase in aging, cancer, and the onset of cardiovascular disease, she draws attention to the links between ongoing stress and illness produced by the wearing down of telomeres:

> [...] what we're finding is that if you don't have good telomerase activity and proper maintenance of telomeres – that actually puts people at risk of cardiovascular disease. The two groups we've got the most immediate data on are care-giver groups – one of which is mothers whose biological child is chronically ill with autism, bowel disease, etc. The mother is the caregiver and she's under stress for not just a short time but years. We found that the worse the stress was and the worse the person perceived it by

quantitative measures, (and you can do that), and the longer she had been in situation, the worse was the wearing down of her telomeres and her risks for developing cardiovascular disease. [...] so there was this possibility that they were literally aging faster. (Hershman Leeson, 2014b)

Dr Blackburn's pioneering work in this field has led to observations that telomerase is active in rapidly dividing cells and is almost universally elevated in cancer patients. A deficiency in telomerase, on the other hand, is associated with a set of bone marrow failure syndromes, while shortened telomeres have been linked to elevated incidences of age-related illnesses, including heart disease. The status of telomeres therefore appears to reflect the health status and risk for chronic diseases in humans, which makes telomere DNA research crucial in a number of fields.

In the interview with Dr Atala, Professor in Regenerative Medicine at Wake Forest, we hear how terminally ill patients can benefit from 3D printed organs. In his work, he notes, children are implanted with the 3D organs that then 'grow and get larger as the children grow'. 'These organs', he continues, 'get identified by the body, as being their own. And they act as if the organs were just the patients' own organ' (interview with Hershman Leeson, 2014c). In answer to Hershman Leeson's question as to whether he was able to transfer or download cells' memories, Atala says:

You know, cells themselves have a memory, so every single cell in your body has all the genetic information to create a whole new you. The idea is you're going to have readymade organs for the patient by using the patient's own cells. The question is, will we be able to have them just on the shelf, ready to put in. In fact, you really could. If you had a bank of organs, which was large enough, you could actually do that. But it's not practical at this point to do so, maybe someday in the future as science evolves. That will become something that will be financially feasible. I may not see it in my lifetime but it's certainly a possibility. (Hershman Leeson, 2014c)

At the heart of Atala's practice is the desire to 'induce the body's own ability to regenerate inside the organ'. Thus, he continues, 'a lot of our efforts right now are aimed towards using the body's own ability to regenerate and to improve that ability'. This can be achieved by programming DNA. Hence, he notes: '[w]e can change the cells' pathway. We can change the cells' fate. We can direct cells from any different directions. The things that we can do with cells today were thought to be entirely science fiction just a few decades ago' (Hershman Leeson, 2014c).

It is evident from these interviews that the 'organ' that is presented in *The Infinity Engine* is one that is intervened with or even produced by biotechnology, and yet it is also an organ that is interfered with whilst it grows inside us, or that is generated outside of us, but is then placed inside of us to become part of us. In the case of Atala's research, the future may even entail a new kind of 'readymade', that is, organs that can be bought off the shelf, commercial products, developed to aid our ability to perform as humans, forming a part of us that may help us to stay alive.

Stasimon: The organic performance framework

Hershman Leeson's practice in *The Infinity Engine* can be described through an organic performance framework. This defines a practice about organisms and organs that emerges through interdisciplinary dialogue, and the positioning of the audience as witness. The practice is about the complex and multifaceted values of life itself in the era in which what it means to be human is being redefined by regenerative medicine. To explain the operation of the organic performance framework, I need to open a parenthesis on certain mechanisms at the heart of the production of scientific knowledge in scientific experimentation. In his influential 1984 paper 'Pump and Circumstance', Steven Shapin points out that 'speech about natural reality is a means of generating knowledge about reality, of securing assent to that knowledge, and of bounding domains of certain knowledge from areas of less specific standing' (1984, 481). In substance, Shapin argues that one of the main resources for validating knowledge within the scientific community was the 'creation of a scientific public' (1984, 481). Using the example of Robert Boyle's experiments in pneumatics in the late 1650s and early 1660s, he shows that Boyle did not only produce new knowledge about the behaviour of air, but also exhibited the means by which 'legitimate knowledge was to be generated and evaluated' (Shapin, 1984, 482). In other words, the production of an experiment involves the identification and dissemination of knowledge about its generation as well as its evaluation to a specific public.

We know that experimentation has a significant rhetorical dimension (Cantor in Gooding et al., 1989, 161) aimed at engaging a public of both experts and non-experts. Shapin, for example, shows that Robert Boyle created a literary form to give prominence to scientific facts wherein the detailed descriptions were meant to encourage the replication of the experiment for the public (1984). The most interesting aspect of Boyle's narrative has therefore to do with the role of the public, since 'seventeenth century scientists often listed the witness present at the experimental trial but Boyle sought through his text to create in the reader the impression of "virtual witnessing" as if the reader had been present in the laboratory' (Cantor in Gooding et al., 1989, 163). Thus the description of an experiment involves the placing of, in this, case, the reader, as a virtual witness to it. In other words, the public must be positioned and even written within the experiment.

But how would the public know whether what they witnessed was true or just opinion? How would they know whether it was fact or spectacle, or both? Shapin points out that three technologies are at work in the establishment of 'matters of fact'. These are: a 'material technology', which in Boyle's case was to do with the operation of the air-pump; a literary technology 'by means of which the phenomena produced by the pump were made'; and 'a social technology that incorporated the conventions experimental philosophers should use in dealing with each other and considering knowledge-claims' (Shapin, 1984, 484). Various 'epistemological strategies' can be used to establish the validity of an experiment which are based on 'looking at the same phenomena with different pieces of apparatus; prediction of what will be observed under specified circumstances;…explanation of observations with an existing accepted theory of the phenomena; the elimination of all sources of error and alternative explanation; calibration and experimental checks;…and statistical validation' (Franklin in Gooding et al., 1989, 21–22). We know that 'experiments are powerful resources for persuasion and conviction' (Gooding et al., 1989, 5). Thus Bruno Latour and Steve Wolgar explain that some of the main elements in creating a laboratory argument are construction, that is, 'the slow, practical craftwork by which inscriptions are superimposed and accounts backed up or dismissed' (1986, 236); agonistic, that is, not so much grounded in nature as in political contention (1986, 237); argument; credibility; circumstances and noise (1986, 237–9). To sum up, three technologies are at stake in the establishment of experimental knowledge, and these are material, literal and societal. For these to be effective, laboratory arguments need to be constructed through epistemological strategies that involve looking at the same data through different perspectives, utilizing accepted existing discourse, and positioning one's argument credibly, but also agonistically in relation to other bodies of knowledge. This, of course, makes laboratory arguments not only rhetorical, but also publicly political.

In *The Infinity Engine,* Hershman Leeson presents a technological process and simultaneous documentation, which is at once material, literary and social. She exhibits the operation of a material technology, 3D printing; introduces aspects of a literary technology, by means of which the practice of 3D printing is made and interpreted; and of a social technology, by incorporating the conventions at stake in dealing with knowledge-claims made possible through 3D printing, including open files of court cases concerning genetic patenting. The public is directly involved in the piece, not only as witness to the event, but also as part of an experiment, which asks of them to participate via their own DNA. Epistemologically, strategies are adopted that allow the public not only to look at, learn from, but also experience the same technology from different points of view, for example, that of a patient as well as that of the medical researcher and the historian of science.

We have already seen that Hershman Leeson frequently uses replication as well as the multiplication of viewpoint in her work. For her in fact:

doubling and tripling was for me a scientific approach in the work. If you could prove something several times, there would be a factor of validity. So, for instance, when we had three Robertas in addition to the original one, their experiences contributed towards the understanding of what Roberta's own experiences meant. The number three constitutes the proof of validity of an assumption. I am told that in science you have to prove something three times. Hence we have three rooms, three Roberta's, three cyborgs, and three critics. (interview with Giannachi, 2008)

Hershman Leeson often utilizes different disciplinary perspectives, 'whether as a psychologist, sociologist, anthropologist, painter', and her practice consists of 'taking elements and collaging them through remixing, creating something that morphs into something beyond itself' (in Giannachi, 2010, 233). This capability of the work to draw from other works, replicate and give birth to new works, is a first distinctive feature of the 'organic' performance framework.

Hershman Leeson works interdisciplinarily, at the cutting edge between science and art. This means that she uses scientific methods to generate art and that her art, in turn, operates through scientific strategies that can produce scientific knowledge. This is particularly noticeable in terms of the relationship between her creation of art as an experience and the possible generation of evidence. The two terms are inter-related. Thus we know that, historically, the term experience 'encompassed a wide range of activities in scientific discourse', and that, for example, 'in the language of medieval natural philosophy, *experientia* and *experimentum* described "tried and proven remedies" that authenticated knowledge through proof' (Findlen, 1996, 203). The *experiential*, which was frequently advocated by Aristotle in his studies of nature (1996, 203–4), in the early modern period, however, became also *evidence* (1996, 204, original emphasis). *The Infinity Engine*, like other works by Hershman Leeson, is also about surveillance and biopolitics, only that here we see 'surveillance from the inside out' (Giannachi, 2014). This capability of the work to constitute at once an experience and to generate evidence is a second distinctive feature of the 'organic performance' framework. This also explains the popularity of the 'Private I' theme in Hershman Leeson's broader body of work, which, in Hershman Leeson's own words, manifests itself in a longing for privacy and visibility that is publicly witnessed in its occurrence as performance (see Hershman Leeson, in Tromble and Hershman Leeson, 2005, 14).

A number of artists have been developing work in the field of bio-art, or bio-media whose practice is significant in this context. One of them is Eduardo Kac who, inspired by the cloning of Dolly the sheep in 1996, followed by the cloning of mice and cows in 1998, started to experiment with genetic engineering to create transgenic art (2005, 236). For Kac, who created a transgenic rabbit, *GFP Bunny* (2000), 'the nature of this new art is defined not only by the birth and growth of a new plant or animal but above all by the nature of the relationship among artist, public, and transgenic organism' (2005, 236–7). The creation of a set of relations between artistic and scientific methodologies and a public, that is often positioned within the experience, as a witness to the generation of a body of evidence, is a third distinctive feature of the 'organic performance' framework. In the case of *The Infinity Engine* the public literally builds knowledge as they proceed through the various bodies of knowledge of the installation to find that they themselves have become part of a growing live archive.

Other artists utilized design and biology to experiment with bio-art from an ontological point of view. For example, Stelarc's *Extra Ear* (1997) was a soft prosthesis built out of cartilage, described as 'a kind of internet antenna that telematically and acoustically scales up one of the body's senses' (Grzinic, 2002, 31). Working in collaboration with SymbioticA, based at the School of Anatomy and Human Biology at the University of Western Australia, Stelarc subsequently took *Extra Ear* a step further. SymbioticA had been producing semi-living tissue, as did the Tissue Culture and Art Project which started in 1996 and for which artists Oron Catts and Ionat Zurr used tissue engineering as a medium for artistic expression to design 'semi-living objects' and 'designed biological objects'. The collaboration led to *Extra Ear ¼ Scale* (2003–2004) that used human cells as a ¼ replica of Stelarc's own ear. This development of art that is not only live, but 'alive' is a fourth distinctive feature of the 'organic performance' framework. Thus in *The Infinity Engine* we witness the exhibition of the scaffolding of a 3-D printed 'nose' that is used at the Wake Forest Center for Regenerative Medicine.

A company whose aesthetic plays a significant role in the conception of *The Infinity Engine* is Critical Art Ensemble, which was also the subject of Hershman Leeson's film *Strange Culture* (2007). The documentary focused on the case of artist and academic Steve Kurtz, a member of Critical Art Ensemble, who, after his wife Hope died of heart failure, was accused on suspicion of bioterrorism by the FBI under the Patriot Act. The company is known for the

creation of participatory performative environments combining a
'cellular practice' (Critical Art Ensemble, 1996, 69) with a digital
aesthetics characterized by copying, which for them consists of
'a process that offers dominant culture minimal material for
recuperation by recycling the same images, actions, and sounds into
radical discourse' (Critical Art Ensemble, 1996, 77), an operation
akin to that of morphing discussed by Hershman Leeson above. In
their *Flesh Machine* (1997–1998) Critical Art Ensemble introduced
themselves as BioCom, a company whose mission was building a
better organic platform for the planet and presented themselves as
a leader in genomics able to advise on reproduction, demonstrating
that 'a "better baby" (one better adapted to the imperatives of pan-
capitalism) can be produced through rationalized intervention'
(Critical Art Ensemble, 2004). Likewise in *GenTerra* (2001–2003)
they presented themselves as a trademarked company, Gentess,
adopting transgenic solutions for a greener world. Participants
could decide whether to activate a transgenic bacteria release
machine that allowed them to prepare samples for their own use
and walk off with a sample of 'recombinant bacteria' containing
a complete random human genome library. For them, 'confusion
should be seen as an acceptable aesthetic' precisely because 'the
moment of confusion is the pre-condition for the skepticism
necessary for radical thought to emerge' (in Meikle, 2002, 132).
The attempt to generate confusion, or dis-orientation, which in *The
Infinity Engine* is achieved through the juxtaposition of different
disciplinary perspectives, is a strategy that is very much akin to
Bertolt Brecht's *Verfremdung* (1961), is a fifth distinctive feature of
the 'organic performance' framework.

Finally, a number of artists, especially women artists, have been
working, since the 1970s, with skin as a *topos* for performance or
even, in the case of ORLAN, for theatre. These include Valie Export,
Alba d'Urbano, Gina Pane, Marina Abramovic and Lynn Hershman
Leeson among others. From their practice it is clear that artists have
been moving away from the eighteenth-century idea of skin as a
boundary between inside and outside, as well as the nineteenth-
century understanding of skin as 'a place of passage to the inside'
(Benthien, 2002, 10–11), and the twentieth-century interpretation
of skin as an interface (Hauser, 2008), instead turning skin into a
site for the curation of 'live' practices. These have been medical,
or aesthetic, or both. The growing importance of skin as a site for

scientific, artistic, political and social intervention, in other words, the identification of skin, or, more broadly, the body as a site for a bio-politically-driven aesthetic, as is clearly shown in *The Infinity Engine,* is a sixth distinctive feature of the 'organic performance' framework.

We know from Michel Foucault that 'the control of society over individuals is not conducted only through consciousness or ideology, but also in the body' through bio-politics, the politics that control 'the biological, the somatic, the corporeal' (1994, 210), for it, in the words of Michael Hardt and Antonio Negri, is about the 'production and reproduction of *life itself*' (Hardt and Negri, 2000, 24, added emphasis). We also know from Donna Haraway that between the First World War and the early 1990s, biology was transformed from 'a science centered on organisms, understood in functionalist terms, to a science studying automated technological devices, understood in terms of cybernetic systems' and that this meant that biology was transformed from a 'science of sexual organisms to one of reproducing genetic assemblages' (1991, 45). Finally, we know from Sarah Franklin that this has had the implication that nature has become biology and then genetics, 'through which *life itself* becomes reprogrammable information' (2000, added emphasis). For her, our DNA results in marketable brand names so that our genes become our capital. The re-definition of life itself, which is at the heart of Hershman Leeson's *The Infinity Engine,* is a sixth distinctive feature of the 'organic performance' framework.

Exode: An after-thought on postmodernism

To sum up, I have suggested that Hershman Leeson's practice presents distinctive features that I wish to describe through an 'organic performance' framework. I have chosen the term 'organic' to indicate that *The Infinity Engine* like other works by Hershman Leeson, is a practice about organisms and organs – in this sense, it is also a medical practice or, to be more precise, a regenerative medical practice. I have chosen the term 'framework' to suggest that this practice is underpinned by a scaffolding mechanism that entails a number of distinctive features. First, the work is often composite and draws from other works and disciplines, often biology, medicine and chemistry, as well as human computer interaction, art, theatre and performance. Unlike the work of other artists who use bio-media, bio-art and transgenic art, Hershman Leeson's project though is not about 'a part of a single work', but rather endeavours to offer 'a complete overview' (Giannachi, 2014). Second, the work frequently constitutes a rich and diverse experience and in the course of this experience evidence is generated that may be significant for a number of parties. Third, the public plays a central role in the work, often acting as witness to the production of meaning through juxtapositions of sets of relations (between scientific facts and fiction; between the voices of different stakeholders, etc.). Fourth, this juxtaposition between different elements is usually not synthesized by the artist. This may cause disorientation or *Verfremdung*, which in turn, politicizes the piece, as it asks of the viewer that they make choices and take up a position. Finally, organic performance is bio-political because it is about life itself, and it addresses its ontological, medical, economic, social, religious, personal, scientific and aesthetic values. Operating interdisciplinarily, this practice draws a number of fundamental strategies from scientific experimentation. First, it involves the identification and dissemination of knowledge about process as well as its evaluation, and possibly documentation of, for a specific public. Second, it entails the placing of the public as participant to, but also as witness of an experience. Third, it involves technologies, which are material, literal and societal and the construction of laboratory arguments through relational epistemological strategies that have rhetorical, as well as political significance. These factors suggest that this practice is both an art *and* a science.

The 'organic performance' framework shows that we have moved beyond the modernist/post-modernist dichotomy identified by Hassan (1982, 269) into a new era, which, typically, retains characteristics of both, but also has a number of distinctive qualities. I have, provocatively, called this era Regeneration, as there are points of comparison with the Renaissance, and I wanted to signal the importance that regenerative medicine is likely to have in all spheres of life. The choice of the term aims to draw attention to the importance of the suffix 're', for in this era we re-play, re-enact, re-cycle, re-store, re-interpret, etc., as well as to the role of generational processes, such as the creation of post-humans, cyborgs, clones, 3D prints, as well as the transmission of our legacy to the next generation. Below, I revisit Hassan's well-known table in the aftermath of these considerations:

Modernism	Postmodernism	Regeneration
Romanticism/ Symbolism	Pataphysics/Dadaism	Performance/ Technology
Form (conjunctive, closed)	Antiform (disjunctive, open)	Process
Purpose	Play	Experience
Design	Chance	Copy/cut/paste
Hierarchy	Anarchy	Biopolitics
Mastery/Logos	Exhaustion/Silence	Training/embodiment
Art Object/ Finished Work	Process/Performance/ Happening	Documentation/ Archive
Distance	Participation	Engagement
Creation/Totalization	Decreation/ Deconstruction	Re-play/Re-enactment
Synthesis	Antithesis	Juxtaposition
Presence	Absence	Mixed Reality
Centring	Dispersal	Emergent
Genre/Boundary	Text/Intertext	Programme/virus
Semantics	Rhetoric	Science
Paradigm	Syntagm	Code
Hypotaxis	Parataxis	Paratactic
Metaphor	Metonymy	Trademark
Selection	Combination	Convergence
Root/Depth	Rhizome/Surface	Internet/skin
Interpretation/ Reading	Against Interpretation/ Misreading	Tagging/Finding
Signified	Signifier	Algorithm
Lisible (Readerly)	*Scriptable* (Writerly)	*Performable* (Practiced)

(Continued)

Modernism	Postmodernism	Regeneration
Narrative/*Grande Histoire*	Anti-narrative/*Petit Histoire*	*Verfremdung*/Hybrid Media
Master Code	Idiolect	DNA
Symptom	Desire	Fever
Type	Mutant	Modified
Genital/Phallic	Polymorphous/Androgynous	Hybrid/Genetic
Paranoia	Schizophrenia	Anxiety
Origin/Cause	Difference-Difference/Trace	Remediated/Network
God the Father	The Holy Ghost	The post-human
Metaphysics	Irony	Prosumption
Determinacy	Indeterminacy	Simulation
Transcendence	Immanence	Co-presence

There have been many calls to the end of post-modernism. Linda Hutcheon, for example, whose 1988 book *A Poetics of Postmodernism: History, Theory, Fiction* has been a standard text, now suggests that the movement may be over (2002). Hassan, himself in his paper, 'Beyond postmodernism: toward an aesthetic of trust' (2003) states that we may have moved beyond the movement, as does Charles Jencks, whose 1977 book *The Language of Post-Modern Architecture* had helped to popularize the term. Thus arguably, as Jeremy Green notes, 'declarations of postmodernism's demise have become a critical commonplace' (2005, 19–24). A number of new theories have since emerged proposing that we are now 'altermodern', shaped by economic globalization and subsequent mass-migration (Bourriaud, 2009); 'hypermodern', living in a society dominated by 'hyperconsumption' (Lipovetsky and Charles, 2005); caught in 'performatism' (Eshelman, 2008); living in an 'automodernity', in between digital automation and personal autonomy (Samuels, 2008); in a technologically run world, in 'digimodernism' (Kirby, 2009). Between them, they range across art and architecture, information technology and the Internet, sociology, film, television and literature. They all acknowledge the role of technology and the global digital economy as well as the impacts of these factors on the human subject. Distinctively, I propose that we still are in the postmodern, but that we attempt to regenerate ourselves from it. The twenty-first-century post-human subject that much of this art attempts to re-present, re-perform, re-cycle, re-play is still experiencing the postmodern 'condition' (Lyotard, 1979), and hence its body is still that of a patient, a medical body, but it is one that is being regenerated inside out, on the edge of a new possible world.

Hershman Leeson's *The Infinity Engine* is a complex work. It is at once a time-based installation, as well as a film, an experiment, evidence and a live archive. It offers multiple disciplinary viewpoints, and it offers multiple aesthetic viewpoints, or ways of entering, engaging with, and even remembering the work (or being remembered in the work). Not unlike Charles Babbage's *The Difference Engine* (1821), an automatic mechanical calculator designed to tabulate polynomial functions based on the method of finite differences, this engine is also about labour, the very labour of life. Myles Jackson points out, whilst talking about *The Difference Engine,* that Babbage's work should challenge us to think about: '[w]hat was the status of manual labor *vis à vis* intellectual labor? Could intellectual skill be mechanized as an ever-increasing set of manual skills could?' For him, questions concerning the management of such labour are dependent on whether that labour was communicable and, if so, how we communicate knowledge to future scientists, engineers and commercial firms, is crucial. For Jackson, in fact '[t]he politics of labor can offer insights into how these issues were solved then and into how those solutions affect decisions being made today' (2013). Hershman Leeson's work too raises questions about labour and its communication, for example, what is the labour of life now that our organs can be regenerated? Who will be benefit from this labour? How can this labour be communicated? As Jackson notes, 'humans are evolving very rapidly, more rapidly than in any other period in history, precisely because of molecular biology and biomedical research' (in Hershman Leeson, 2013c). Hershman's work presents us for the first time with a complex and experimental analysis of what these processes of regeneration and evolution may entail for us.

NOTES

Introduction

1 For example, the MSc in Medical Humanities at Kings College London targets 'medical and health professionals; students of health policy; those who wish to pursue further academic study in medicine and/ or the humanities … and [those] considering careers in journalism or bioethics'. We are including bordering disciplines such as medical sociology, the sociology of health and illness and the history of medicine within this.

2 Academic departments concerned with performance practices come under a variety of titles (e.g. Drama, Theatre, Dance, Performance, Performing Arts) and these can have very different remits in terms of the art-forms studied and pedagogic approaches (skills-based practical training; academic study and combinations of the two).

Chapter 1

1 To see Dion discussing the process around this project see: http:// narratingwaste.wordpress.com/2010/05/04/mark-dion-and-tate-thames- dig-1999-an-extract/. For other Cabinet works by Dion also see Sheedy.

2 Abreu, J. (2014), *Blood*, Performance at Rich Mix, London, 25 January 2014.

3 For more information on this production see Abreu's website: http://www.jeanabreudance.com/ (accessed 1 September 2014).

4 Shaw, P. and Weaver, L., *RUFF*, performance at the Bristol Old Vic Studio, 16 May 2014.

Chapter 2

1 See especially Jane R. Goodall (2003), *Performance and Evolution in the Age of Darwin*, London: Routledge.

2 Kirsten E. Shepherd-Barr (2015), *Theatre and Evolution from Ibsen to Beckett*, New York: Columbia University Press.

3 See Chapter 7, 'Doctors' Dilemmas', in Shepherd-Barr, K. (2006), *Science on Stage: From Doctor Faustus to Copenhagen*, Princeton: Princeton University Press.

Chapter 3

1 'The Social', *chchsocial.tumblr.com* http://chchsocial.tumblr.com/ [accessed 19 June 2014].
2 'The Integratron Is the fusion of Art, Science and Magic', *Integratron .com* http://integratron.com/about/ [accessed 19 June 2014].
3 'The Spa Ethos', *rotoruamuseum.co.nz* http://www.rotoruamuseum .co.nz/things-to-see-and-do/taking-thecure/the-spa-ethos/ [accessed 19 June 2014].

Chapter 4

1 The piece was piloted at the 2012 Cheltenham Literature Festival and premiered at the South Asian Dance Summit (Bournemouth) and The Place (London) in 2013.

Chapter 5

1 This is explored literally in Lobel's later work *An Appreciation* where audience members are invited to medically 'appreciate', i.e. handle his genitals.
2 Documentation of Flanagan's performance work is included in the documentary *Sick: The Life and Death of Bob Flanagan, Supermasochist* dir. Kirby Dick (1997).
3 Shown in the Santa Monica Museum of Art in 1992–1993, the New Museum in New York City in 1994 and the Museum of Fine Arts in Boston in 1995.
4 First presented by Dixon Place, New York, as part of PS122's Coil Festival in 2013.
5 A company that Shaw founded alongside Lois Weaver (long-time collaborator and co-writer and director of *RUFF*) and Deb Margolin.
6 Both Lobel's *BALL* and Shaw's *Must* have been presented as part of Clod Ensemble's 'Performing Medicine' programme which uses arts in medical education.

Chapter 8

1 A prime example of this in the UK is Eyam in Derbyshire. In 1665, 260 people in the village died from the plague which was started by a tailor ordering a bale of cotton from London. In an act of self-sacrifice the inhabitants sealed off the village to prevent the plague from spreading further.

Chapter 9

1 For more detailed historical accounts of the birth of dissection see, for example, F. French (1999), *Dissection and Vivisection in the European Renaissance*, Aldershot: Ashgate; A. Cunningham (1997), *The Anatomical Renaissance*, Aldershot: Scolar Press; and A. Carlino (1999), *Books of the Body: Anatomical Ritual and Renaissance Learning*, trans. J. & A. Tedeschi, Chicago & London: University of Chicago Press.
2 See Clod Ensemble's website for further details of their work and projects: http://www.clodensemble.com
3 These names are listed as such in the programme notes for the piece.
4 See, for instance, C. Waldby & R. Mitchell (2006), *Tissue Economies: Blood, Organs and Cell Lines in Late Capitalism*, London & Durham: Duke University Press; and J. Gareth & M. I. Whitaker (2009), *Speaking for the Dead: The Human Body in Biology and Medicine*, Farnham & Burlington: Ashgate.
5 For more information on the legal situation and its implications, see D. Dickenson (2007), *Property in the Body: Feminist Perspectives*, Cambridge: Cambridge University Press; and R. Hardcastle (2009), *Law and the Human Body: Property Rights, Ownership and Control*, Oxford & Oregon: Hart Publishing.

Chapter 10

1 See M. Kemp and M. Wallace (2000), *Spectacular* Bodies, London: Hayward Gallery and D. Petherbridge and L. Jordanova (1998), *The Quick and The Dead*, Los Angeles: University of California Press.

Chapter 11

1 These incidents took place during, or after, visits to abattoirs near Sydney (2011), Dublin (2013) and Ljubljana (2013), respectively, whilst procuring fresh pig hearts for live perfusion performances for

The Body is a Big Place installation. Hearts were obtained as a by-product of abattoir processing: no animals were harmed for the direct purpose of the performances.

Chapter 12

1   21 April 2014. This can be viewed here: https://www.youtube.com/watch?v=uKXzwBly_Ak

2   A more developed version of the project, staged at the *Medicine in Motion* event at Chisenhale Dance Space in London, UK (January 2015), used an elegant and simple device for overcoming this issue of exposition. The resulting performances by a range of people with experiences of chronic pain prompted empathetic and enthusiastic audience responses.

3   J. Abreu, *Blood* project webpage: http://www.jeanabreudance.com/tours/blood [accessed 16 February 2015].

4   Itze Maître, website on *The Primary Intimacy of Being*: http://www.lepixelblanc.co/primary-intimacy-of-being/ [accessed 16 February 2015].

5   C. Djeressi (2002), *An Immaculate Conception,* full English-language text available at www.djerassi.com/icsi/immaculate.doc [accessed 16 February 2015].

6   Dublin Science Gallery webpage on the Semi-Living Worry Dolls. Available at: https://dublin.sciencegallery.com/visceral/semi-living-worry-dolls/ [accessed 16 February 2015].

7   Visceral exhibition website, including film: http://www.symbiotica.uwa.edu.au/activities/exhibitions/visceral [accessed 16 February 2015].

8   This emphasis on the 'live' is my justification for including sculptures within a chapter on performance. I'm supported in this by Sally Jane Norman's 'Anatomies in Live Art' in Anatomy Live which draws attention to the bioreactor as a sort of stage.

9   Kathy High, 'Blood Wars' video accompanying *Visceral* exhibition: https://www.youtube.com/watch?v=wBmtEp7sutU [accessed 16 February 2015].

10   Https://www.youtube.com/watch?v=wBmtEp7sutU

BIBLIOGRAPHY

Agamben, G. (1994), 'The Cabinet of Wonder', in *The Man Without Content*, trans. G. Albert, California: Stanford University Press.

Aitkenhead, D. (1999), 'Unprivate Lives', *The Guardian*, 28 June, p. 15.

Alberti, S. M. M. (2011), *Morbid Curiosities: Medical Museums in Nineteenth Century Britain*, Oxford and New York: Oxford University Press.

Anderson, B. (1991), *Imagined Communities: Reflections on the Origin and Spread of Nationalism*, London and New York: Verso.

Anker, S. and Nelkin, D. (2004), *The Molecular Gaze: Art in the Genetic Age*, New York: Cold Spring Harbour Laboratory Press.

Appelbaum, D. (1990), *Voice*, Albany: State University of New York Press.

Arends, B. and Thackara, D. (1999), *Experiment: Conversations in Art and Science*, London: The Wellcome Trust.

Australian and New Zealand Intensive Care Society (2010), *The ANZICS Statement on Death and Organ Donation*, Edition 3.1. www.anzics.com.au/death-and-organ-donation [accessed 20 July 2014].

Bakhtin, M. (1984), *Rabelais and His World*, trans. H. Iswolsky, Indianapolis: Indiana University Press.

Barilan, Y. M. (2004), 'Medicine Through the Artist's Eyes', *Perspectives in Biology and Medicine*, 47, pp. 110–134.

Barrow, K. and Jackson, T. (2010), 'Picture Your Life After Cancer', *The New York Times Online*. http://www.nytimes.com/interactive/2010/04/08/health/cancer-survivor-photos.html?ref=health [accessed 9 February 2015].

Bates, V. and Bleakley, A. (2013), *Medicine, Health and the Arts*, London and New York: Routledge.

Bates, V., Bleakley, A. and Goodman, S. (2014), *Medicine, Health and the Arts: Approaches to the Medical Humanities*, Abingdon & New York: Routledge.

Baudrillard, J. (1983), *Simulations*, trans. P. Foss, P. Patton and P. Beittchman, New York: Semiotex[e].

Baudrillard, J. (1998; [1970]), *The Consumer Society*, trans. C. Turner, London: Sage Publications.

Bayly, S. (2011), *A Pathognomy of Performance*, Basingstoke: Palgrave Macmillan.

Benedict, B. M. (2001), *Curiosity: A Cultural History of Early Modern Inquiry*, Chicago and London: University of Chicago Press.

Benjamin, W. (1999), *The Arcades Project*, R. Tiedemann (ed), trans. H. Eiland and K. McLaughlin, Harvard: Harvard University Press.

Benthien, C. (2002), *Skin: On the Cultural Border between Self and the World*, New York: Columbia University Press.

Bernat, J. L. (2007), 'Reply by James L. Bernat, MD', in Steinberg, D. (ed), *Biomedical Ethics: A Multidisciplinary Approach to Moral Issues in Medicine and Biology*, Hanover and London: University Press of New England, p. 85.

Bleeker, M. (2011), *Visuality in the Theatre: The Locus of Looking*, Basingstoke: Palgrave Macmillan.

Bouchard, G. (2012), 'Skin Deep: Female Flesh in Live Art since 1999', *Contemporary Theatre Review*, 22(1), pp. 94–105.

Bourriaud, N. (2009), 'Altermodern'. http://www.tate.org.uk/whats-on/tate-britain/exhibition/altermodern [accessed 5 August 2014].

Braidotti, R. (2002), *Metamorphoses: Towards a Materialist Theory of Becoming*, Cambridge: Polity Press.

Brecht, B. (1961; [1936]), 'On Chinese Acting', trans. E. Bentley, *The Tulane Drama Review*, 6(1), pp. 130–136.

Brodzinski, E. (2010), *Theatre in Health and Care*, Basingstoke, Hampshire and New York: Palgrave Macmillan.

Campbell, A. (2009), *The Body in Bioethics*, London and New York: Routledge.

Campos, L. (2013), 'Science in Contemporary British Theatre: A Conceptual Approach', in Bartleet, C. and Shepherd-Barr, K., 'New Directions in Theatre and Science Part 1', *Interdisciplinary Science Reviews*, December 2013, 38 (4), pp. 295–303.

Carlson, M. (2001), *The Haunted Stage: The Theatre as Memory Machine*, Ann Arbor: University of Michigan Press.

Cartwright, L. (1995), *Screening the Body: Tracing Medicine's Visual Culture*, Minneapolis: University of Minnesota Press.

Cole, T., Carlin, N. and Carson, R. (2014), *Medical Humanities: An Introduction*, Cambridge and New York: Cambridge University Press.

Cork, R. (2012), *The Healing Presence of Art: A History of Western Art in Hospitals*, New Haven and London: Yale University Press.

Critical Art Ensemble (1996), *Electronic Civic Disobedience*. http://critical-art.net [accessed 11 January 2014].

Critical Art Ensemble (2004), *BioCom*. http://www.critical-art.net/biotech/biocomWeb/product.html [accessed 11 January 2014].

Crouch, Tim (2011a), *Plays One*, London: Oberon, pp. 38–39.

Crouch, T. (2011b), *Tim Crouch: Plays One*, London: Oberon Books.

Cunningham, A. (2010), *The Anatomist Aantomis'd: An Experimental Discipline in Enlightenment Europe*, Farnham: Ashgate.

Cushing, N. and Markwell, K. (2010), 'I Can't Look: Disgust as a Factor in the Zoo Experience' in Warwick, F. (ed), *Zoos and Tourism: Conservation, Education, Entertainment?*, Bristol: Channel View Publications, pp. 167–178.

Davenne, C. (2011), *Cabinets of Wonder*, New York: Abrams.

Davis, L. J. (2009), *Biocultures*. www.leanarddavis.com/biocultures.html [accessed 10 July 2014].

Davis, L. J. and Morris, D. B. (2009), *Biocultures Manifesto*. www.leanarddavis.com/biocultures.html [accessed 10 July 2014].

De Beer, G. (ed) (1983), *Charles Darwin and T.H. Huxley: Autobiographies*, Oxford: Oxford University Press.

Dean, B. (2011), 'Endings and Beginnings', Catalogue essay for *The Body Is a Big Place* installation, Performance Space, Sydney.

DeVita, M. A. and Arnold, R. M. (2007), 'The Concept of Brain Death', in Steinberg, D. (ed), *Biomedical Ethics: A Multidisciplinary Approach to Moral Issues in Medicine and Biology*, Hanover and London: University Press of New England, pp. 82–85.

Dieckmann, P., Gaba, D. and Rall, M. (2007), 'Deepening the Theoretical Foundations of Patient Simulation as Social Practice', *Simulation in Healthcare*, 2(3), pp. 183–193.

Dion, M. (2010), 'Mark Dion and "Tate Thames Dig" (1999) – An Extract' in Waste Effects'. http://narratingwaste.wordpress.com/2010/05/04/mark-dion-and-tate-thames-dig-1999-an-extract/ [accessed 1 September 2014].

Djerassi, C. (1998), *An Immaculate Conception*. www.djerassi.com/icsi/immaculate.doc [accessed 7 December 2014].

Dumit, J. (2012), 'Prescription Maximization and the Accumulation of Surplus Health in the Pharmaceutical Industry', in Sunder Rajan, K. (ed), *Lively Capital: Biotechnologies, Ethics and Governance in Global Markets*, Durham and London: Duke University Press.

Ede, S. (2000), 'Many Complex Collisions: New Directions for Art in Science', in Ede, S. (ed), *Strange and Charmed: Science and the Contemporary Visual Arts*, London: Calouste Gulbenkian Foundation.

Ede, S. (2010), *Art and Science*, London: Tauris

Ehrenreich, B. (2009), *Bright-Sided: How the Relentless Promotion of Positive Thinking Has Undermined America*, New York: Metropolitan Books.

Elkins, J. (1996), *The Object Stares Back: On the Nature of Seeing*, New York and London: Harcourt Brace and Co.

Eshelman, R. (2008), *Performatism, or the End of Postmodernism*, USA: The Davies Group Publishers.

Evans, M. and Finlay, I. (2001), *Medical Humanities*, London: British Medical Journal.

Featherstone, M. and Burrows, R. (1995), *Cyberspace, Cyberbodies, Cyberpunk*, London: Sage.

Ferrari, G. (1987), 'Public Anatomy Lessons and the Carnival: The Anatomy Theatre of Bologna', *Past and Present*, No. 117 (November), Oxford: Oxford University Press, pp. 50–106.

Findlen, P. (1996; [1994]), *Possessing Nature: Museums, Collecting, and Scientific Culture in Early Modern Italy*, Berkeley: University of California Press.

Flanagan, B. and Rose, S. (1997), 'Performance Art: (Some) Theory and (Selected) Practice at the End of This Century', *Art Journal*, 56(4), pp 58–59.

Foucault, M. (1970), *The Order of Things: An Archaeology of the Human Sciences*, New York: Routledge Classics.

Foucault, M. (1978), *A History of Sexuality: Volume One, an Introduction*, trans. R. Hurley, New York: Pantheon Books.

Foucault, M. (1994), 'La Naissance de la medicine sociale', *Dits et écrits*, 3, Paris: Gallimard.

Foucault, M. (1999; [1973]), *The Birth of the Clinic: An Archaeology of Medical Perception*, trans. Sheridan, A. M., New York: Routledge Classics.

Frank, A. W. (1991), *At the Will of the Body: Reflections on Illness*, New York: Mariner Books.

Frank, A. W. (1995), *The Wounded Storyteller: Body, Illness and Ethics*, Chicago: University of Chicago Press.

Franklin, S. (2000), 'Life Itself: Global Nature and the Genetic Imaginary', in Franklin, S., Lury, C. and Stacey, J. (eds), *Global Nature, Global Culture*, London: Sage.

Fraser, A and M. Greco (2005), *The Body: A Reader*, London and New York: Routledge.

Freud, S. (1916), 'Some Character-Types Met with in Psychoanalytic Work,' in vol. 14 of *The Standard Edition of the Complete Psychological Works*, 24 vols., ed. and trans. Strachey, James. London: Hogarth Press, 1953–1974.

Freud, S. (1925), 'Some Character-Types Met with in Psycho-Analytic Work', in *The Standard Edition of the Complete Psychological Works of Sigmund Freud*, Strachey, J. (ed), *vol. XIV (194–1916): On the History of the Psycho-Analytic Movement, Papers on Metapsychology and Other Works*, London: Hogarth Press.

Furse, A. (2006), 'Performing in Glass: Reproduction, Technology, Performance and the Biospectacular', in Harris, G. and Aston E. (eds), *Feminist Futures? Theatre, Performance, Theory*, Basingstoke and New York: Palgrave Macmillan, pp. 149–168.

Gallego, J. (2014), 'The Dissector's Cut, the Wound and the Orifice. Seeing Ron Athey's Performances through a Cultural Anatomy of the Vagina', *Performance Research*, 'On Medicine', 19(4), pp. 74–84.

Garland-Thompson, R. (2006), *Staring: How We Look*, Oxford: Oxford University Press.

Garland-Thompson, R. (2009), 'From Wonder to Error', in Blanchard, P. et al. (eds), *Human Zoos: Science and Spectacle in the Age of Colonial Empires*, Liverpool: Liverpool University Press.

Garner, Jr., S. B. (2008), 'Is there a Doctor in the House? Medicine and the Making of Modern Drama', *Modern Drama* 51(3) (Fall), pp. 311–328.

Giannachi, G. (2008), interview with Lynn Hershman Leeson, San Francisco. Private archive.

Giannachi, G. (ed) (2010), 'Lynn Hershman Leeson in Conversation with Gabriella Giannachi', *Leonardo*, 43(3), pp. 232–233.

Giannachi, G. (2014), Interview with Lynn Hershman Leeson, San Francisco. Private archive.

Gilbert, W. S. (1870), *A Medical Man. Drawing-Room Plays and Parlour Pantomimes*, collected by C. Scott from E.L. Blanchard [and others], London.

Gilbert, M., Busund, R., Skagseth, A., Åge Nilsen, P. and Solbø, J. P. (2000), 'Resuscitation from Accidental Hypothermia of 13.7°C with Circulatory Arrest', *The Lancet*, 355, pp. 375–376.

Gillespie, B. (2013), 'Ruff by Peggy Shaw and Lois Weaver (Review)', *Theatre Journal*, 65(4), 576–577.

Gladstone, M. and J. C. Berlo (2011), 'The Body in the (White) Box: Corporeal Ethics and Museum Representation', in Marstine J. (ed), *The Routledge Companion to Museum Ethics*, London and New York: Routledge.

Goffman, E. (1959), *The Presentation of Self in Everyday Life*, London: Penguin.

Goodall, J. R. (2003), *Performance and Evolution in the Age of Darwin*, London: Routledge.

Gooding, D., Pinch, T. and Schaffer, S. (eds) (1989), *The Uses of Experiment: Studies in the Natural Sciences*, Cambridge: Cambridge University Press.

Gotman, K. (2010), 'Vertigo', in Willson, S. and P. Clark, *Clod Ensemble: Under Glass*, Programme Notes.Available from www.clodensemble. com – Clod Ensemble, 2-18 The Laundry, London E8 3FN.

Gray, C. H. (2002), *Cyborg Citizen: Politics in the Posthuman Age*, London and New York: Routledge.

Green, J. (2005), *Late Postmodernism: American Fiction at the Millennium*, New York: Palgrave.

Griffith, S. (2014), 'Mirror, Mirror on the Wall – Who Has the Fairest ORGANS of Them All?', *Daily Mail*, 17 April 2014. http://www.dailymail. co.uk/sciencetech/article-2606779/Mirror-mirror-wall-fairest-ORGANS-Smart-surface-reveals-insides.html [accessed 16 February 2015].

Grosz, E. (1994), *Volatile Bodies: Toward a Corporeal Feminism*, Bloomington and Indianapolis: Indiana University Press.

Grzinic, M. (ed) (2002), *Stelarc*, Ljubljana, Maribor: Maska.

Hannah, D. (2007), 'Containment + Contamination: A Performance Landscape for the Senses at PQ03', in Banes, S. and Lepecki, A. (eds), *The Senses in Performance*, New York and Oxon: Routledge, pp. 135–145.

Haraway, D. (1991), *Simians, Cyborgs, and Women: The Reinvention of Nature*, London: Free Association Books.

Hardt, M. and Negri, A. (2000), *Empire*, Cambridge, Massachusetts: Harvard University Press.

Hassan, I. (1982; [1971]), *The Dismemberment of Orpheus: Toward a Postmodern Literature*, Madison: University of Wisconsin Press.

Hassan, I. (2003), 'Beyond Postmodernism: Toward an Aesthetic of Trust', in Stierstorfer, K. (ed), *Beyond Postmodernism: Reassessments in Literature, Theory and Culture*, Berlin: de Gruyter, pp. 199–212.

Hauser, J. (ed) (2008), *Sk-Interfaces: Exploding Borders – Creating membranes in Art, Technology and Society*, Liverpool: Fact and Liverpool University Press.

Heddon, D. (2007), *Autobiographical Performance: Performing Selves*, Basingstoke: Palgrave Macmillan.

Hershman Leeson, L. (1996), *Clicking In: Hot Links to a Digital Culture*, Seattle, WA: Bay Press.

Hershman Leeson, L. (2013a), '*The Infinity Engine*: a Live Cinematic Installation', production brochure, private archive.

Hershman Leeson, L. (2013b), *The Infinity Engine*. http://www. theinfinityengine.com/lynn.html [accessed January 2014].

Hershman Leeson, L. (2013c), *The Infinity Engine*. https://www. kickstarter.com/projects/theinfinityengine/the-infinity-engine-lab [accessed 10 August 2014].

Hershman Leeson, L. (2014a), 'The Infinity Engine Installation Footprint', Hershman Leeson private archive.

Hershman Leeson, L. (2014b), Lynn Hershman Leeson's interview with Elizabeth Blackburn, Hershman Leeson private archive.

Hershman Leeson, L. (2014c), Lynn Hershman Leeson's interview with Antony Atala, Hershman Leeson private archive.

Hill, L. and Paris, H. (2014), *Performing Proximity: Curious Intimacies*, Basingstoke: Palgrave.

Holroyd, M. (1989), *Bernard Shaw vol. 2: 1898–1918, The Pursuit of Power*, London: Chatto and Windus.

Hooper Greenhill, E. (1992), *Museums and the Shaping of Knowledge*, London: Routledge.

Hunsaker Hawkins, A. (1999), *Reconstructing Illness: Studies in Pathography*, West Lafayette: Perdue Research Foundation.

Hutcheon, L. (1989), *The Politics of Postmodernism*, London and New York: Routledge.

Hutcheon, L. (2002), 'Postmodern Afterthoughts', *Wascana Review of Contemporary Poetry and Short Fiction*, 37(1), pp. 5–12.

Jackson, A. (2007), *Theatre, Education and the Making of Meanings: Art of Instrument?*, Manchester: Manchester University Press.

Jackson, M. (2013), 'Charles Babbage on Intellectual and Manual Skill', *The Huffington Post*. http://www.huffingtonpost.com/myles-jackson/charles-babbage-on-intell_b_2760780.html [accessed 10 August 2014].

Jaffe, T., 'Peggy Shaw "Ruff"', *Front Row Center*. http://thefrontrowcenter.com/2014/01/919/ [accessed 1 April 2014].

Jencks, C. (1977), *The Language of Postmodern Architecture*, Milano: Rizzoli.

Jennings, S. (1997), *Dramatherapy with Families, Groups and Individuals: Waiting in the Wings*, London and New York: Routledge.

Jones, H. A. (1897), *The Physician: An Original Play*, London: re-printed by Kessinger Publishing, Montana (in 2010).

Jones, A. (1998), *Body Art: Performing the Subject*, Minnesota: University of Minnesota Press.

Jones, A. and Warr, T. (eds) (2012), *The Artist's Body*, London: Phaidon Press.

Kac, E. (2005), *Telepresence and Bio Art*, Ann Arbor: The University of Michigan Press.

Kassab, E., Kyaw Tun, J. and Kneebone, R. (2012), 'A Novel Approach to Contextualized Surgical Simulation Training', *Simulation in Healthcare: Journal of the Society for Simulation in Healthcare*, 7, no. 3: doi:10.1097/SIH.0b013e31824a86db.

Kassab, E., Kyaw Tun, J., Arora, S., King, D., Ahmed, K., Miskovic, D., Cope, A. and others (2011), '"Blowing Up the Barriers" in Surgical Training: Exploring and Validating the Concept of Distributed Simulation.' *Annals of Surgery*, 254, no. 6: doi:10.1097/SLA.0b013e318228944a.

Kauffman, L. (1998a), *Bad Girls and Sick Boys: Fantasies in Contemporary Art and Culture*, Berkeley: University of California Press.

Kauffman, L. (1998b), 'Sadomedicine: Bob Flanagan's "Visiting Hours" and Last Rites', *Performance Research*, 3(1), pp. 32–40.

Kemp, M. (2006), *Seen/Unseen: Art, Science, and Intuition from Leonardo to the Hubble Telescope*, Oxford: Oxford University Press.

Kemp, M. and Wallace, M. (2000), *Spectacular Bodies*, London and Los Angeles: Hayward Gallery and University of California Press.

Kirby, A. (2009), *Digimodernism: How New Technologies Dismantle the Postmodern and Reconfigure Our Culture*, London: Bloomsbury Academic.

Kirshenblatt-Gimblett, B. (1998), *Destination Culture: Tourism, Museums, and Heritage*, London and Los Angeles: University of California Press.

Kneebone, R. (2009), 'Perspective: Simulation and Transformational Change: The Paradox of Expertise', *Academic medicine: Journal of the Association of American Medical Colleges*, 84(7), pp. 954–957.

Kneebone, R. (2010), 'Simulation, Safety and Surgery', *Quality and Safety in Health Care*, 19(Ergonomics and Safety Supplement), pp. i47–i52.

Kneebone R. (2011), 'The art, science and simulation of performance', *International Symposium on Performance Science*. Toronto.

Kneebone R. (2014), 'Escaping Babel: The Surgical Voice', *The Lancet*, 384, pp. 1179–1180.

Kneebone, R. and Williamon, A. (2013), *The Scalpel and the Bow*. 30 minute radio feature. BBC Radio 3: BBC.

Kneebone, R., Arora, S., King, D., Sevdalis, N., Kassab, E., Aggarwal, R., Darzi, A. and Nestel, D. (2010), 'Distributed Simulation – Accessible Immersive Training', *Medical Teacher*, 32(1), pp. 65–70.

Kracauer, S. (1992), 'Abschied von der Lindenpassage', in Rosenberg, V. J. (ed), *S. Kracauer: Der verbotene Blick*. Leipzig: Reclam, 49–55.

Krpic, T. (2014), 'The Politics of Intimate Medical Performances: Ive Tabar's body-art performances El-en-I and Acceptio', *Performance Research*, 'On Medicine', 29(4), pp. 64–73.

Kuppers, P. (2003), *Disability and Contemporary Performance: Bodies on Edge*, London and New York: Routledge.

Kuppers, P. (2004), 'Visions of Anatomy: Exhibitions and Dense Bodies', *Differences: A Journal of Feminist Cultural Studies*, 15, pp. 3.

Kuppers, P. (2007), *The Scar of Visibility: Medical Performances and Contemporary Art*, Minneapolis: University of Minnesota Press.

Kuppers, P. (2014), *Studying Disability Arts and Culture: An Introduction*, Basingstoke: Palgrave Macmillan.

La Fleur, W. R. (1990), 'Hungry Ghosts and Hungry People: Somacity and Rationality in Medieval Japan', in Feher, M., Naddaff, R. and Tazi, N. (eds), *Fragments for a History of the Human Body Part One*, Massachusetts and London: MIT Press.

Langley, D. (2006), *An Introduction to Dramatherapy*, London, California and New Delhi: Sage Publications.

Latour, B. and Wolgar, S. (1986; [1979]), *Laboratory Life: The Construction of Scientific Facts*, Princeton: Princeton University Press.

Leder, D. (1990), *The Absent Body*, Chicago: University of Chicago Press.

Lewes, G. H. (1875), *On Actors and the Art of Acting*, London: Smith, Elder and Co.

Lipovetsky, G. and Charles, S. (2005), *Hypermodern Times*, Cambridge: Polity Press.

Llubljansko barje visitor information. http://www.ljubljanskobarje.si/en/
ljubljana-moors/waters [accessed 16 February 2015].

Lobel, B. (2012a), *BALL and Other Funny Stories About Cancer*,
London: Oberon Books.

Lobel, B. (2012b), *CancerCancerCancerCancerCancer, collected cancer
works by Brian Lobel*, London: Live Art Development Agency, DVD.

Lobel, B., Jansen, C. and Okubo, N. (2013), *Fun with Cancer Patients*.
http://www.funwithcancerpatients.com [accessed 15 February
2015].

Lupton, D. (2012), *Medicine and Culture: Illness, Disease and the Body*,
London, California and New Delhi: Sage Publications.

Lyotard, J. F. (1984), *The Postmodern Condition: A Report on
Knowledge*, trans. G. Bennington, B. Massumi and F. Jameson,
Minneapolis: University of Minnesota Press.

Lyotard, J.-F. (1985 [1979]). *The Postmodern Condition*. Tr. G.
Bennington and B. Massumi. Manchester: Manchester University Press.

Lyotard, J.-F. (1988), *The Differend, Phrases in Dispute*, trans. G. van den
Abbeele, Minneapolis: University of Minnesota Press.

MacDougall J. and Yoder, P. S. (eds) (1998), *Contaminating Theatre:
Intersections of Theatre, Therapy and Public Health*, Illinios:
Northwestern University Press.

Malkin, J. R. (1999), *Memory-Theatre and Postmodern Drama*, Ann
Arbor: University of Michigan Press.

Mamet, D. (1998), *Three Uses of the Knife*, London: Methuen.

Mauriès, P. (2002), *Cabinets of Curiosities*, London: Thames and
Hudson.

McConachie, B. (2008), *Engaging Audiences: A Cognitive Approach to
Spectating in the Theatre*, Basingstoke: Palgrave Macmillan.

McConachie, B. (2012), *Theatre and Mind*, Basingstoke: Palgrave
Macmillan.

McConachie, B. and Hart, E. (2006), *Theatre and Cognition: Theatre
Studies and the Cognitive Turn*, London and New York: Routledge.

Meikle, G. (2002), *Future Active: Media Activism and the Internet*,
London and New York: Routledge.

Menninghaus, W. (2003), *Disgust: Theory and History of a Strong
Sensation*, New York: State University of New York Press.

Miller, I. (2014), *Colliding Worlds: How Cutting-Edge Science in
Redefining Contemporary Art*, New York: W.W. Norton and
Company.

Moraru, C. (2012), 'Contagion, Contamination, and Don Delillo's
Post-Cold War World-System: Steps toward a Haptical Theory of
Culture', in Magnusson, B. and Zalloua, Z. (eds), *Contagion: Health,
Fear, Sovereignty*, Washington: University of Washington Press and
Whitman College, pp. 123–148.

Morley, D. and Chen, K-H. (eds) (1996), *Stuart Hall: Critical Dialogues in Cultural Studies*, New York: Routledge.

Morrison, H. (2013), 'Conversing with the Psychiatrist: Patient Narratives Within Glasgow's Royal Asylum, 1921–29', *Journal of Literature and Science*, 6(1), pp. 18–37. http://www.journalofliteratureandscience.org [accessed 14 January 2014].

Mukherjee, S. (2011a), 'Should We Stop Trying to Cure Cancer?', *Guardian Weekend*, 5 January 2011.

Mukherjee, S. (2011b), *The Emperor of All Maladies: A Biography of Cancer*, London: Fourth Estate.

Multerud, K (2001), 'The Art and Science of Clinical Knowledge: Evidence Beyond Measures and Numbers', *The Lancet*, 358(9279), pp. 379–400.

Nestel, D. and Bearman, M. (eds) (2014), *Simulated Patient Methodology: Theory, Evidence, and Practice*, Chichester: Wiley-Blackwell.

Newman, H. (2004), 'Connotations', in Heathfield, A. (ed), *Live: Art and Performance*, London: Tate Modern, pp. 166–175.

Ngai, S. (2005), *Ugly Feelings*, Cambridge: First Harvard University Press.

Nicholson, H. (2014; [2009]), *Applied Drama: The Gift of Theatre*, Basingstoke: Palgrave Macmillan.

Norman, S-J. (2008), 'Anatomies of Live Art', in Bleeker, M. (ed), *Anatomy Live: Performance and the Operating Theatre*, Amsterdam: Amsterdam University Press.

Nussbaum, M. (2004), *Hiding from Humanity: Disgust, Shame, and the Law*, New Jersey: Princeton University.

O'Brien, M. (2012), 'Abject Clearances: Considering the Cough, Mucus and Breathing', in Keidan, L. and Mitchell, C. J. (eds), *Access All Areas: Live Art and Disability*, London: Live Art Development Agency, pp. 89–91.

O'Casey, S. (1985), *Seven Plays by Sean O'Casey: A Students' Edition*, R. Ayling (ed), London: Macmillan.

O'Reilly, S. (2009), *The Body in Contemporary Art*, London: Thames and Hudson.

Oswald, A. (2010), 'The Village', in Willson, S. and P. Clark, *Clod Ensemble: Under Glass*, Programme Notes available from www.clodensemble. com – Clod Ensemble, 2-18 The Laundry, London E8 3FN.

Park-Fuller, L. (2008), 'How to Tell a True Cancer Story', *Text and Performance Quarterly*, 28, pp. 178–182.

Parker-Pop, T. (2010), 'Picture Your Life After Cancer', *The New York Times Online*. http://well.blogs.nytimes.com/2010/04/08/picture-your-life-after-cancer/ [accessed 15 February 2015].

Parker-Starbuck, J. (2011), *Cyborg Theatre: Corporeal/Technological Intersections in Multimedia Performance*, Basingstoke: Palgrave.

Parnia, S. (2007), 'Do Reports of Consciousness During Cardiac Arrest Hold the Key to Discovering the Nature of Consciousness?', *Medical Hypotheses*, 69, pp. 933–937.

Parry, J. (2013), Review of Jean Abreu's *Blood*, 1 July 2013, DanceTabs. http://dancetabs.com/2013/07/jean-abreu-dance-blood-london/ [accessed 16 February 2015].

Paul, H. W. (2011), *Henri de Rothschild, 1872–1947: Medicine and Theater*, Farnham, Surrey: Ashgate.

Pearce, S. M. (1994), 'Collecting Reconsidered', in Pearce, S. M. (ed) *Interpreting Objects and Collections*, London: Routledge.

Petherbridge, D. and Jordanova, L. (1997), *The Quick and the Dead: Artists and Anatomy*, London: National Touring Exhibitions.

Petros, P. (2001), 'The Art and Science of Clinical Knowledge', *The Lancet*, 358(9295), pp. 1818–1819.

Pettit, F. (2012), 'The Afterlife of Freak Shows', in Kember, J., Plunkett, J. and Sullivan, J. A. (eds), *Popular Exhibitions, Science and Showmanship, 1840–1910*, London: Pickering and Chatto.

Phelan, P. (1997), *Mourning Sex: Performing Public Memories*, London and New York: Routledge.

Pogue Harrison, R. (1992), *Dominion of The Dead*, Chicago: University of Chicago Press.

Popa, V. (2011), *Vasko Popa: Complete Poems 1953–1987*, trans. A. Pennington and F. R. Jones, London: Anvil Press Poetry.

Poyatos, F. (1993), *Nonverbal Communication Across Disciplines: Paralanguage, Kinesics, Silence, Personal and Environmental Interaction*. Amsterdam: John Benjamins Publishing Co.

Pynor, H. (2014), Email correspondence with Mermikides. Private archive

Qureshi, S. (2004), 'Displaying Sara Baartman, the "Venus Hottentot"', *History of Science*, 42 (June),pp. 233–257.

Qureshi, S. (2011), *Peoples on Parade: Exhibitions, Empire, and Anthropology in Nineteenth-Century Britain*, Chicago: University of Chicago Press.

Quick, A. (2007), *The Wooster Group Workbook*, New York: Routledge.

Renza, L. (1972), 'The Veto of the Imagination: A Theory of Autobiography', in Olney, J. (ed), *Autobiography*, Princeton: Princeton University Press.

Richardson, R. (2000), *Death, Dissection and the Destitute*, London and Chicago: University of Chicago Press.

Rogers, B. (2012), 'Unwrapping the Past: Egyptian Mummies on Show', in Kember, J., Plunkett, J. and Sullivan, J. A. (eds), *Popular Exhibitions, Science and Showmanship, 1840–1910*, London: Pickering and Chatto.

Rosenthal, K. (2011). 'Everything Changes Blog'. http://everythingchangesbook.com/ [accessed 15 February 2015].

Roy, S. (2009), 'Clod Ensemble', *The Guardian*, 13 May 2009. http://www.
theguardian.com/stage/2009/may/13/review-clod-ensemble [accessed
10 February 2015].

Samuels, R. (2008), 'Auto-Modernity after Postmodernism: Autonomy
and Automation in Culture, Technology, and Education', in
McPherson, T. (ed) *Digital Youth, Innovation, and the Unexpected*,
Cambridge, MA: The MIT Press, pp. 219–240.

Sandahl. S. and Auslander, P. (2005), *Bodies in Commotion: Disability
and Performance*, Ann Arbor: University of Michigan Press.

Sawday, J. (1995), *The Body Emblazoned: Dissection and the Human
Body in Renaissance Culture*, London: Routledge.

Scarry, E. (1985), *The Body in Pain: The Making and Unmaking of the
World*, New York and Oxford: Oxford University Press.

Schechner, R. (2013; [2002]), *Performance Studies: An Introduction*,
London: Routledge.

Schwartz, H-P. and Shaw, J. (1996), *Perspektive der Medienkunst*,
Karlsruhe ZKM: Cantz Verlag.

Schweizer, H. (2002), 'The Question of Meaning in Suffering',
Unpublished conference paper delivered at Making Sense of Health,
Illness and Disease. St. Catherine's College, Oxford.

Shapin, S. (1984), 'Pump and Circumstance: Robert Boyle's Literary
Technology', *Social Studies of Science*, 14, pp. 485–520.

Shaughnessy, N. (2012), *Applying Performance: Live Art, Socially
Engaged Theatre and Affective Practice*, Basingstoke: Palgrave
Macmillan.

Shaughnessy, N. (2013), *Affective Performance and Cognitive Science:
Body, Brain and Being*, London: Bloomsbury Methuen Drama.

Shaviro, S. (1995), 'Two Lessons from Borroughs', in Halbertstam, J.
and Livingston, I. (eds), *Post-Human Bodies*, Bloomington: Indiana
University Press, pp. 38–56.

Shaw, B. (1897), 'Ghosts at the Jubilee', *Saturday Review*, 2 July 1897,
pp. 12–14.

Shaw, G. B. (1906), *The Doctor's Dilemma. The Complete Plays of
Bernard Shaw*. London: Odhams Press, 1934.

Shaw, B. (1934), 'The Doctor's Dilemma', in *The Complete Plays of
Bernard Shaw*, London: Odhams Press.

Shaw, P. and Weaver, L. (2014), RUFF performance at the Bristol Old Vic
Studio, 16 May 2014.

Sheedy, C. J. (ed) (2006), *Cabinet of Curiosities: Mark Dion and the
University as Installation*, Minneapolis: University of Minnesota
Press.

Sheets-Johnstone, M. (2009), *The Corporeal Turn: An Interdisciplinary
Reader*, Exeter and Charlottesville: Imprint Press.

Shepherd-Barr, K. (2006), *Science on Stage: From Doctor Faustus to Copenhagen*, Princeton and Oxford: Princeton University Press.

Shepherd-Barr, K. (2015), *Theatre and Evolution from Ibsen to Beckett*, New York & Chichester: Columbia University Press.

Shildrick, M. (2008), 'Contesting Normative Embodiment: Some Reflections on the Psycho-social Significance of Heart Transplant Surgery', *Perspectives: International Journal of Philosophy*, 1, pp. 12–22.

Showalter, E. (1987), *The Female Malady: Women, Madness and English Culture, 1830–1980*, London: Penguin Books.

Silverman, L. (2012), 'Social Media Help Diabetes Patients (and Drugmakers) Connect', 3 December 2012. http://www.npr.org/blogs/health/2012/12/03/166241115/social-media-helps-diabetes-patients-and-drugmakers-connect [accessed 1 February 2014].

Snow, R., Humphrey, C. and Sandall, J. (2013), 'What Happens When Patients Know More than their Doctors? Experiences of Health Interactions after Diabetes Patient Education: A Qualitative Patient-led Study.' *BMJ Open*, 3(11) pp. 1–9 (online).

Sparling, K. (2005), 'About' Six Until Me'. http://sixuntilme.com/wp/about-kerri-sparling/ [accessed 1 February 2014].

Sparling, K. (2007), '*Your Story*' in Six Until Me http://sixuntilme.com/yourstory/ [accessed 1 February 2014].

Sparling, K. (2011), 'You Are More Than Diabetes', 26 September 2011. http://sixuntilme.com/wp/videos/ [accessed 1 February 2014].

Sparling, K. (2012a), 'Diabetes Burnout', 22 January 2012. http://sixuntilme.com/wp/videos/ [accessed 1 February 2014].

Sparling, K. (2012b), 'Kerri's OneTouch Ping Story', 13 September 2012. http://sixuntilme.com/wp/videos/ [accessed 1 February 2014].

Sparling, K. (2012c), 'The Proof Is in the People', 31 December 2012. http://diatribe.org/issues/50/sum-musings [accessed 1 February 2014].

Sparling, K. (2014), 'Complications', 11 June 2014. http://sixuntilme.com/wp/page/2/ [accessed 14 June 2014].

Sparling, K. and Edelman, S. (2013), 'Meet OneTouch VerioIQ Guides', 3 January 2013. http://sixuntilme.com/wp/videos/ [accessed 1 February 2014].

Spence, J. (1986), *Putting Myself in the Picture: A Political Personal and Photographic Autobiography*, London: Camden Press.

Stacey, J. (1997), *Teratologies: A Cultural Study of Cancer*, London and New York: Routledge.

Stacey, J. (2010), *The Cinematic Life of the Gene*, Durham and London: Duke University Press.

Stafford, B. (1993), *Body Criticism: Imaging the Unseen in Enlightenment Art and Medicine*. Cambridge, MA: The MIT Press.

Stahl, D. (2013), 'Living in the Imagined Body: How Diagnostic Image
    Confronts the Lived Body', *The British Journal of Medical Humanities*,
    39(1), pp. 53–58.
Stelarc and Atzori, P. and Woolford, K. (1995), 'Extended-Body: Interview
    with Stelarc' in *CTheory*. http://www.ctheory.net/articles.aspx?id=71.
    [accessed 1 September 2014].
Teresi, D. (2012), *The Undead: Organ Harvesting, the Ice-Water Test,
    Beating Heart Cadavers – How Medicine Is Blurring the Line Between
    Life and Death*, New York: Vintage Books.
Thompson, J. (2009), *Performance Affects: Applied Theatre and the End
    of Effect*, Basingstoke: Palgrave Macmillan.
Tromble, M. and Hershman Leeson, L. (eds) (2005), *The Art and Films
    of Lynn Hershman Leeson: Secret Agents, Private I*, Berkeley: The
    University of California Press.
Turner, V. (1995), *The Ritual Process: Structure and Anti-Structure*,
    London: Aldine.
Twigger, R. (2010), *Angry White Pyjamas: A Scrawny Oxford Poet Takes
    Lessons from the Tokyo Riot Police*, London: HarperCollins.
Vanden-Hauvel, M. (2013), 'The Acceptable Face of the Unintelligible:
    Intermediality and the Science Play', in Bartleet, C. and Shepherd-
    Barr, K. (eds), 'New Directions in Theatre and Science Part 1',
    Interdisciplinary Science Reviews, December, 38 (4), pp. 365–379.
Van Dijck, J. (2005), *The Transparent Body: A Cultural Analysis of
    Medical Imaging*, Washington: University of Washington Press.
Vergine, L. (2000), *Body Art and Performance*, Milan: Skira.
Vitruvius (1914), *The Ten Books on Architecture*, trans. M. Hicky
    Morgan, Cambridge MA: Harvard University Press.
Waddington, K. and Willis, M. (2013), 'Introduction: Rethinking
    Illness Narratives', *Journal of Literature and Science*, 6(1),
    pp. iv–v. http://www.journalofliteratureandscience.org [accessed 14
    January 2014].
Warren, J. (2008), 'Performing Trauma: Witnessing *BALL* and the
    Implications for Autoperformance', *Text and Performance Quarterly*,
    28, pp. 183–187.
White, G. (2015), *Applied Theatre Aesthetics*, London, New Delhi, New
    York and Sydney: Bloomsbury Methuen Drama.
Wilkinson, S. (2013), Review of Jean Abreu's 'Blood', *The Stage*. http://
    www.thestage.co.uk/reviews/review.php/38704/blooddated28June
    2013 [accessed 16 February 2015].
Willis, M., Waddington, R. and Marsden, R. (2013), 'Imaginary
    Investments: Illness Narratives Beyond the Gaze', *Journal of Literature
    and Science*, 6(1), pp. 55–73. http://www.journalofliteratureandscience.
    org [accessed 14 January 2014].

Wilson, E. A. (2004), *Psychosomatic: Feminism and the Neurological Body*, Durham and London: Duke University Press.

Wilson, S. (2012), *Science + Art Now: How Scientific Research and Technological Innovation Are Becoming Key to Twenty-First Century Aesthetics*, London: Thames and Hudson.

Willson, S. and P. Clark (2010), *Clod Ensemble: Under Glass*, Programme Notes.

Winship, L. (2013), feature on Jean Abreu's 'Blood', *Time Out*, 25 June 2013. http://www.timeout.com/london/dance/gilbert-george-and-jean-abreu-get-blood-on-the-dancefloor [accessed 16 February 2015].

Wolff, T. (2009), *Mendel's Theatre: Heredity, Eugenics, and Early Twentieth-Century American Drama*, London: Palgrave Macmillan.

Woods, A. (2013), 'Rethinking "Patient Testimony" in the Medical Humanities: The Case of Schizophrenia Bulletin's First Person Accounts', *Journal of Literature and Science*, 6(1), pp. 38–54. http://www.journalofliteratureandscience.org [accessed 14 January 2014].

Zola, E. (1978), 'Naturalism in the Theatre', preface to *Thérèse Raquin*, reprinted in Worthen, W. B. (ed.), *Modern Drama: Plays, Criticism, Theory*. Boston: Harcourt Brace, 1994. pp. 1179–1187.

Zola, E. (1995), 'Naturalism in the Theatre', trans. A. Bermel, in Worthen, W. B. (ed), *Modern Drama: Plays/Criticism/Theory*, Texas: Harcourt Brace College Publishers, pp. 1182–1186.

INDEX